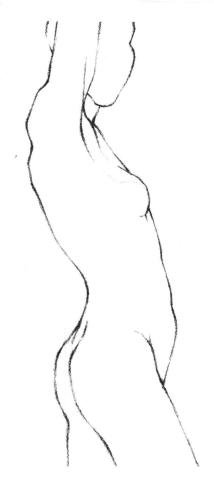

Twenty-Something & Breast Cancer
"IMAGES IN HEALING"

Twenty-Something & Breast Cancer

"IMAGES IN HEALING"

IN PRINT PUBLISHING
Sedona, Arizona

IN PRINT PUBLISHING

Published by
IN PRINT PUBLISHING
6770 West Highway 89A, #46
Sedona, Arizona 86336

Artwork on title page by Mary Phelan
Design and layout by Blaine Fairchild

Preassigned LCCN: 9576-50

Manufactured in the United States of America
by Griffin Printing, Sacramento, CA

ACKNOWLEDGMENTS

My deepest thank-you goes out to all the people who have helped me live through this experience and write this book...

Tomi Keitlen, for believing in me.

Dr. Arnie Herman, for being a friend and surgeon, as well as planting the seed for this book.

Dr. Rochelle Strenger, Dr. David Barrall, and Dr. Gabrielle Masko, for their honesty, caring, the ability to humor me and respect my thoughts and opinions.

Nurse Diane, for never once missing!

The two most incredible brothers that a girl could ask for, Jeff and Kevin Phelan, for their ever present love and support. Their wives—Linda, for always being available with a strong shoulder, and Mary, for her kind and loving words at all the right moments and her special friendship.

My sister Rosemary, for being able to hold my hand and ease my fears long distance.

My two loyal, furry friends, Kai and Banded.

Beth Trieschmann, for being my sweet angel, caretaker, and dear friend.

Stephen Trieschmann, for sharing his new bride and persuading me to always move on to that next level of running.

Karen Ramos, and Andrea Leonard, for their motherly nurturing.

Donna Ross, whose friendship is the priceless part of the experience.

Carolyn Schmitz, for her love and friendship, as well as her ability to cry!

Mary Ann Silvia, M.S.W. and Dr. Steven Fors, for being able to see beneath my tough exterior and always being available to me.

Laura Buckler, for being my inspiration.

Susan Andrews, for being such a beam of light in my life.

Joanne Braz, for her faith and trust in my character!

My parents, Irma Maria Hasicke Phelan, and Joseph Benidict Phelan, for giving me life.

Rosie Boyle, Kim Longo, Lyn Fors, Debbie Lotz, All of the Breast Health Group, Nancy Nelso, Danielle Boule, Kay Jenkins, Paul Bazzoni, Janice Oyer, Janie Esquivel, Linda and Niki Smith, Donna Marie Spencer, Collette Fortin, Robin Rodgers, Darlene Fleury, Leslie Keene, Denise Lach, Paul Boule, Leslie Barker, and all the loving, supportive friends and clients I may have missed.

Juliet Wittman, for taking time out for a total stranger.

Patricia Staebler, for her gift.

The entire Breast Friends Group; Jill Roche, Donna Ross, Arlene McAuley, Ronni Neckes, Lynn Carter, Susan Peterson, Joy Veaudry, Susan Ricci, Mary D'Esposito, Rene Bentley, Jane Pagano, Mae Mazzeo, and Nancy Winslow.

My daughters, Cara and Meghan, for reminding me to laugh, filling me with endless amounts of bliss and joy, and maintaining my world.

My husband Michael, for his unconditional love, patience and self-sacrificing devotion to me.

And to God, for everything.

DEDICATION

To Cara and Meghan

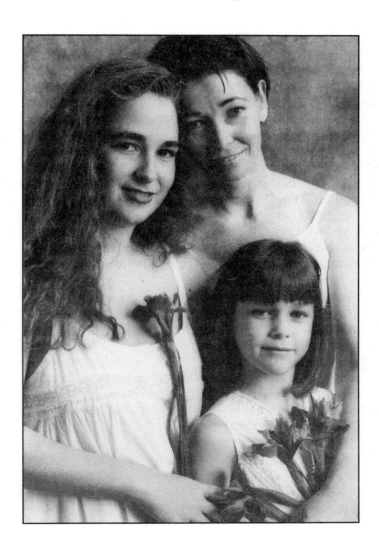

PUBLISHER'S NOTE

The alarming statistics that one woman in eleven will face breast cancer, makes this very personal account both necessary and compelling reading. This book is directed, not only to the women affected by the disease, but to the men in their lives and to their families and friends who are also devastated by the pronouncement,"you have cancer of the breast."

Perhaps, this book will fulfill the need for understanding, for compassion and the need for education in coping with, and, ultimately, helping to find a cure for this dreaded disease.

To preserve the authenticity of the author's experience, the original choice of words and structure have been left virtually intact with only a minimum of changes.

TABLE OF CONTENTS

PREFACE

Reflecting back on my journey through cancer, I realize that it has been almost five years since the diagnosis. I have watched and experienced the four seasons change, gaining some sort of momentum and strength through them all. My writing has not only been extremely therapeutic, but it has also served as a much needed diversion for me. I have only recently decided to go back to the beginning and complete my reflections in hope of publishing the journal of my journey. I feel the need to give back something from my experience, to somehow bring hope and life into the word cancer. But, most of all, to share.

There will be many woman diagnosed with cancer this year, both young and old. Many will do as I have, and search the book stores for encouraging, hopeful reading material, preferably written by another woman who has endured and even been enlightened by this illness. The chances of finding this sort of reading material are slim. There are books, good books, written by M.D.'s, Ph.D.'s, and even nurse practitioners. The question is, "have they had breast cancer?" Women seek and desire other women to share, and learn from. This makes the availability of such material very important.

I hope that any man or woman will be able to pick up this book and gain something positive and strengthening from its words and feelings. My words and emotions are honest. So honest they may at times seem a bit insulting, but understand that this was not my intention. There are parts that some will find very controversial and this is OK too. This is my experience and not everybody who reads about it will be able to identify with it. The words are coming straight from my journal with very few alterations.

I need to say that cancer, or any other illness, does not have to center around pain, and suffering. Not to say that these things won't be experienced because they most certainly will be. This remains a very important part of the healing process. But, these painful and negative emotions should not be the nucleus of the entire experience. We must utilize the experience in a more positive way in order to grow through it. My experience is mostly about love and having the courage to open my heart to the love and growth that I have to share with those around me.

Since we don't ever see things as they are, but rather, as we are, the experience will vary from person to person. So in the situation at hand, whether it be cancer or a gall bladder attack, there always remains a choice. Will the disease bring experiences which will benefit our life, or not. How do we *choose* to experience it?

The flame of the aspiration must be so straight and so ardent that no obstacle can dissolve it.

—The Mother
Pondicherry, India

FOREWORD

This year 182,000 women will be told they have breast cancer. Over 58,000 will be women under fifty years of age. A very precious few will be in their twenties. Each will be forced to deal with the heavy issues of life and death, alterations in their self-image, their relationships with others, and the heavy burden of maximum surgery, chemotherapy, and radiation. All this at a time when their peers are dealing with diapers and the latest fashions.

In this remarkable journal, Linda Phelan McCoy unselfishly shares with us the very personal and internal trauma that breast cancer imposes upon a vital, outgoing, dynamic, and loving woman. The strength that she draws from within herself, her circle of friends and family supplements her deep spiritual faith and trust.

Linda was able to remain in control of her treatments by speaking openly with her physicians and challenging some of their recommendations. She complemented traditional medical therapy with well-researched and balanced alternative therapies. Although many physicians react negatively to an assertive patient that does not capitulate to their treatment plan, more patients need to realize the value of participating in their therapy decisions. Especially since many of the changes in modern cancer therapy come not from the research laboratory, but from the patients themselves.

Her story emphasizes that patients should discuss treatment recommendations with their doctors and question any aspect that is not clear. They should not hesitate to seek a second opinion to confirm the original plan. Libraries, bookstores, local and national cancer societies and telephone hotlines can provide additional information to help make the decisions easier. Only when one is comfortable with the treatment plan can there be the inner peace and acceptance that allows the treatments to proceed without major emotional stresses.

I have learned much from Linda in our previous interactions. The new insights I have gained from this book enable me to understand how I may better meet the needs of my patients. Linda's insights into her journey show us the needs of a woman with breast cancer and the impact that life-threatening disease can have upon her and her family.

Linda's continued joyous celebration of life throughout her treatment allows us to laugh and cry with her. By sharing in her journey, we gain the ability to deal with the adversity in our lives in a positive and productive way.

Arnold Herman, M.D., F.A.C.S.

CHAPTER 1

LOOKING BACK

"Remember this...our world is one where the impossible occurs every-day, and what we often call supernatural is simply the misunderstood."

—Louis L'Amour

At age four, the word *cancer* had little or no meaning for me at all. That was, of course, until I caught my mother crying in the kitchen, wiping the tears with a dish towel. She took me into her room and said, "Linda, there is something that you should know. Your Taunte Hilde has cancer and she is going to die soon."

"Die! Well, why does she have to die? She *is* in a hospital where they make people better, so why does she have to die?"

"Well, because she has had the cancer for a long time now and there is no more that the doctors can do," she replied.

And so it was, my beautiful Aunt died at the young age of 44. From that point on, all I knew was that if you had cancer long enough you were certain to die from it.

There was a ten year age difference between my mother and her sister but it never had any effect on the closeness they shared. After her sister's death, it seemed forever before my mother was normal again. Or at least what we expected to be normal. The only thing in her life that brightened her eyes was flying. She flew gliders as a very young woman in Germany. Her love for flying never diminished. It only intensified through the years. It was her haven, her religion, and her way to be near God. Being the first female flight instructor in New England was something she took great pride in.

Her father, my Opa, had been an aeronautical designer, as well as a concert pianist and zither player. He died from leukemia four years before I made my entrance into this world. My mother absorbed quite a bit of pain and suffering, both from her childhood in a work camp, as well as negative emotions regarding her sister's death. I believe she dreaded following her sister's fate. And so it was...by the time I was twelve years old my mother was diagnosed with breast cancer. The cancer had already made its way into her bones by the time of the diagnosis.

My father, all six foot three inches of him, was at a loss to help her. My parents had such different lives before they met that you had to wonder how they communicated at all. My father was 100% Irish heritage (and proud of it!) with a gruff voice and intense mannerisms. He could have made any room fall silent upon entering it. He first met my mother when she was nineteen years old, in Newport, Rhode Island. She had immigrated there seeking freedom and peace.

I believe she was attracted to him for many reasons, but their age difference was a security for her. He was fifteen years older than she. Although he fathered her in some ways and took very good care of her, he lacked the ability to emotionally support her through cancer. After her diagnosis, he was lost. He made his way through the next two years of hell by reminiscing. When there was that certain sparkle in his eyes I knew he was remembering those very dear memories of her. He would look up at me and say with complete joy, "Linda, I'll never forget the day I first set my eyes upon your mother. She was so striking! At first she wanted nothing to do with me, but eventually I won her over with that indisputable Phelan charm."

Together they had three children. The first was Rosemary, five years older than myself, then Jeffrey, two years older, and myself. I can't deny that I was a Daddy's girl. My mother spent most of her time in airplanes with Jeff. They were so close that at times I wondered if they were "connected" in some way. For two years we watched my mother go through various combinations of crude chemotherapy, radiation, more surgery and so on. She successfully kept her fear, anger and pain well hidden from all of us. It just sat inside her like a ball of cement, waiting for her to fall down from the unbearable weight.

We continued with our yearly, and sometimes twice yearly flights aboard Lufthansa to Germany. Jeff and I had chosen this as our favorite memory of her. We would step off the plane in Stuttgart, turn around, and witness the most extraordinary yet beautiful transformation taking place in her. Her five foot five inch frame, with shining black hair falling against her beautiful pale skin and incredibly dark eyes, stood like a tightly closed rose bud opening up to the perfect day of sun. This was surely her home. My father witnessed this maybe once or twice, which was why he probably chose not to accompany us. I think it made him feel terribly inadequate.

When I was thirteen we made the trip that was to be her last. Once we were home, she attempted to renew her pilot's license. When that was denied, she gave up the fight. I remember that day. I heard her sob uncontrollably in her bedroom. I had never heard that sound before. She was saying, "Why? Why must it be like this? If I cannot fly, then what do I have to live for?"

My mother obviously couldn't figure out the answer to that question, and six months later she was turned into the ground, also at age forty-four. I lay in bed crying, asking God how he could have done this. Why couldn't I have suffered? I reached out my arms to wrap around my father's thick waist in every effort to keep him together. He held, and I looked into his sad green eyes, "Dad, remember, you have always told me that death is a very necessary part of living, and we all must do it to get to the next place."

He cried, "You're absolutely right Linda, but why Irma? Why my beautiful Irma?"

So at age fourteen I forfeited my teenage years so that I could hurry and grow up. I needed to take care of the two men I had left. I bought my first bra and shaved my legs. This was something my mother was completely against, no matter how terribly I got teased by my peers. I sold my horse, and gave up gymnastics. This allowed me way too much time to plant in myself the same ugly seeds of fear my mother had planted in herself. I dreaded the disease.

I tortured myself with the memory of her scarred body. I never saw my mother undressed until one day shortly before her death when I was alone in the house with her. She was in the bathtub when I heard her call my name. I was both stunned and mortified. I waited to see if she would call again and she did. I walked slowly down the hall and grasped the door knob with sweaty palm and turned it ever so gently with my eyes half closed. As I entered the room she handed me a washcloth and in a fragile voice that I barely recognized, asked, "Linda, could you please wash my back since I can no longer reach it myself ?"

I finally had to open my eyes all the way. I nearly fainted at the sight. Who was this woman? My mother was strong and vibrant, nothing like this crippled patchwork quilt sitting before me. For years, I could not understand why she called me in that day. Then I realized that she must have known that she would die soon. She wanted to somehow get started on something we had never attempted to do—establish that beautiful mother-daughter relationship. Something I would only see in other people's lives now. But, rather than remember that moment with grief, I could now remember it with great love. Thinking back on this, I wrote in my journal:

> *"We are not tied to memories for the importance of the memory, but rather for the emotions they hold on to."*

So much took place in the next five years. At age sixteen, I gave birth to a beautiful, healthy baby girl, Cara. Cara Maria, after my mother. She became my world, my vision into the future. Together we would grow, live and learn. But, best of all, we shared that perfect, unconditional love that can only be experienced between mother and child.

My father had retired in California with his widowed sister, my Aunt Marge. I followed, finished high school, then went on to college. I was determined to make it through college on my own. Completely against my father's wishes, I lived apart from him. He would look me square in the eyes and say, "Now Linda, you know that both you and my little shortcake would be much safer and comfortable living here in my home." It never dawned on him that I was a combination of both my parents. This meant that once my mind was set on independence, it was set and I made it work.

My half brother Kevin, whom I adored, joined us later with his wife, Mary, and daughter, Maura. I felt a strong connection to Kevin. He reminded me of my father in a wonderful way. Mary was like a sister to me, when I was fifteen and pregnant as well as later on. She didn't speak much, but her presence did. After graduation, I accepted a job as a dental assistant in Vermont, where I didn't know a soul. We lived there for two years before returning to Rhode Island after the death of my father. I longed for that sense of family once again. I knew that I would be close to my brothers, Jeff, and Kevin when he moved back East.

I met and married my husband, Michael—the complete opposite of the type I'd always said I would marry. In my imagination, I married into a nice big Italian family, ate loads of Italian food, and exchanged good old Italian hugs. No, instead I married quiet, Irish Michael with the face of a little boy. It must have been his silent interaction with Cara that first made me think of long-term commitment with this man. But, then again, his beautiful blue eyes and perfectly slim build helped too! The fact that his family was even smaller than mine concerned me. I really adored the thought of a large family, without thinking of all the hassles and disputes of course!

We married January 5, 1985 and he adopted Cara. She was seven years old. They absolutely adored each other. Cara welcomed her new father with wonderful enthusiasm. Her long thin body would jump up into his arms and smile with beautiful amber eyes. Together, they could light up a sky. A short time later I gave birth to our second daughter, Meghan Beth. I changed careers, going into massage and muscle therapy, when Meghan began having seizures, at two-and-a-half years old.

Meg's illness was more stressful than I could have ever imagined. A brain tumor was ruled out and we began treating the "idiopathic" (of unknown cause) condition with Tegretol. Both Michael and I hated giving it to her since she experienced every side effect imaginable. She would stand in the kitchen and look up at me with those incredible blue eyes and blond curls and ask, "Why do I have to take that Mommy? It makes my belly hurt."

I was jogging to relieve the stress of school and Meg's poor health. It was after a long summer's run one evening that I came home and draped my damp body across our bed, barely conscious. I began to run my hand around my breasts, almost as if being guided by an angel. My breath stopped. I found something. My fingers began to play with this hard, fleshy ball and very quickly I realized what was going on. The little ball was in the very lower portion of my right breast.

I phoned my OB/GYN only to find that he was in Turkey. His office recommended I make an appointment with our family practitioner. I was seen within days and from there referred to a surgeon. He was a large man with those specs that seem to stare down at you. I thought, just let me know what the hell this thing was. We discussed my family history while he attempted to aspirate (draw a sample out through a needle) the lump. When that failed he said, "Just bear with me for a few more minutes while I obtain a cell biopsy." I thought it was odd that there was no nurse in the room to comfort me during this very uncomfortable procedure but didn't argue with the man when he proceeded to jab several needles into my tender breast.

He finished and looked up at me again, " I am certain that this is absolutely nothing, but I will order a sonogram and do a little arguing with the radiologist to get him to perform a mammography. They don't like to do them in such young, healthy women. I won't need to see you again, but you should make an appointment with your OB/GYN for a follow-up and I will send him all the necessary information and reports. Here is a book I would like to lend you. I think you should read it and become familiar with the signs of a *real* breast problem. By the way, what was your mothers name?"

"Irma Phelan."

" I was her surgeon," he replied. "By the time I opened her up it was already in her bones so I referred her to my brother in law who is an oncologist." *Terror* was the best word I could find to describe my emotion.

I followed up with my regular doctor and he confirmed that all was fine. I questioned having the lump removed for sanity's sake. The doctor told me, "There is no need to mark up your breasts Linda. It is only a cyst." Mike was with me and supported my concern, but he was undeniably relieved with the doctors words. By December the "cyst" had grown and I was sitting in my new office with a friend and client. She felt the lump and agreed I should telephone the doctor.

The receptionist answered and I said, " Hello there, this is Linda McCoy. The doctor examined me in July for a cyst and I would like to speak to him about my concern that it is growing."

"The doctor is busy, but I will relay your message to him and get back to you within the half hour." So we sat and waited. She phoned back, "The doctor wants me to tell you to *relax*. It is simply a cyst and they can get larger or smaller. Enjoy the holidays and we will see you in the Spring for your annual pap smear and exam."

I suppose part of me was relieved. As directed, I arrived in Spring for my exam. Upon reexamining the right breast, the doctor replied, "Still cystic." Mike had joined me to lend emotional support since I had decided again to pursue the idea of having the lump removed. The doctor spoke to my husband, "In Turkey the women have every little lump removed due to a lack of sophisticated techniques such as mammography, and their breasts become uneven and unattractive. There is absolutely no reason for Linda to consider this procedure."

We left, a bit numb, forced to be content with his words. After all, this was the man I trusted to deliver my daughters. That was, until the dreaded day in June when I was watching a movie and reached up to scratch an itch on the upper portion of my left breast. My heart began to race uncontrollably when my hand landed upon a small pealike lump. I swear, an angel must have tickled me.

I phoned my doctor and he ordered another mammography. There was no time to ask Michael to meet me there since it all happened so fast. The doctor examined my breast and informed me that, again, the mammography was normal. He attempted to aspirate it with no luck. By then I was in tears. He looked at me with those condescending eyes and said, "Linda if you are going to be so ridiculous over this new little cyst, I will send you over to the emergency room and have a resident remove it with some local anesthesia." Not even a mention of the right breast "cyst" which by this time was the size of a half dollar. I cried all the way home and for the first time in my years of seeing him, I decided to go elsewhere for another opinion.

A horse woman friend of mine gave me the telephone number of one of her best friends, Karen, who had just completed chemotherapy for breast cancer. I barely made it through the door when I grabbed the phone and dialed. She was so supportive and sympathetic, almost as though she knew something I didn't. "Oh, you poor thing," she said. "You're only twenty-nine and you have to deal with all of this." We ended the conversation and Karen gave me the name and number of a reputable breast surgeon in Providence. She was leaving for a trip to Europe with her husband to celebrate her triumph, but promised to phone me when she got home. Karen seemed like a real life guardian angel.

I phoned Dr. Arnold Herman's office the next day. I liked his name. It sounded very strong. His receptionist, Pat, could not have been more accommodating or kind, and made an appointment for me to be seen that week. I was nervous yet grateful.

Although I had no idea who my guardian angel was, I knew I wanted her here with me. Something told me that it was her mission to guide me. She had reached a higher level of existence herself through her disease, and now she was earning her wings by extending compassion toward another. But, she was visible to me. I could talk to her and hear her voice in response. I could touch her, and she could hold my hand. This, too, was a lesson. I was learning to *believe*.

CHAPTER 2

JOURNEYING THROUGH THE INNER

    I spoke to Michael about the new appointment and he listened contentedly. "Linda, you need peace of mind and this is what you need to do to get it." He seemed relieved that I was going several steps further with this, but at the same time he refused to think that it could be anything life threatening. It seemed the doctor's brainwashing had taken effect on him. I worried that he would be in denial if it turned out to be anything but a cyst.

    Anxiously I entered Dr. Herman's office, but I soon felt a profound sense of calmness. I must have been in the right office. The energy felt strong, yet peaceful. Pat greeted me," Linda— relax, sit down and fill out this health history form." She showed me into a small library filled with books and a television. "I'm going to put on a tape. It is just standard. Something we ask all of our new breast patients to watch. I'll be back in a few minutes." I reviewed all the books on the shelf. They were all about breast cancer. I felt myself begin to sweat. Just then Pat opened the door, "It's your turn." I sighed, then took a deep breath and went in.

    I was barely into my gown when Dr. Herman presented himself. He conveyed a positive presence as a very intuitive and tactful person. He slid my mammography films on the viewer and said, "I can't see anything on the left film, but here (circling the site of the right breast mass) is the mass in the right breast."

I had to catch my breath, "I was told that nothing showed up on these films." He did not respond, and I felt terribly uncomfortable that I had put him on the spot.

He slid his glasses down and looked at me, "I believe that both masses are one of the same thing, whatever they may be. Your concern is valid. You have a strong family history. I think we should set up an appointment to remove them both and get a better look at them." I was grateful that he said 'we'. I felt so alone in the past with hearing 'me, me, me', and 'you'!

We discussed the problems with using mammography as a diagnostic tool in younger women. Dr. Herman said that mammography was less effective due to the density of the breast tissue, so we must rely more on direct examination. He explained the only safe way to deal with the situation was to remove the two lumps. I was relieved that someone was finally taking a serious interest in my health. There was concern in his voice regarding my ominous family history, and I admitted that the thought frightened me.

Dr. Herman seemed confident, but not cocky. He respected what I had to say and never appeared to be in a rush, quite the opposite. We spent as much time talking about my profession as we did my health. He was very interested in a course I had recently completed in Toronto, Canada called Manual Lymphatic Drainage (MLD). It was a technique designed by a husband and wife medical team to more efficiently treat various forms of edema. Dr. Herman had several patients who underwent radical mastectomy surgery twenty or so years ago, and now experienced a problem with edema. He admitted that he had always felt like a part of the puzzle was missing. We agreed to discuss it further at another time convenient for us both.

I was relieved the biopsy surgery wouldn't cost me more than one day of work. I had just moved into a larger office space and hired another therapist named Deborah. I had a problem of always feeling the need to be in control, and was not too happy with the thought of someone else running my business. Deb said, "Linda, don't worry. You'll be back here in no time and if I have any problems I'll be sure to find you." I hadn't known her very long, yet I felt in my heart that I could trust her.

My surgery date was scheduled. It was only 12 short days away. I had a lot of explaining to do before then. I was terrified to let my brother, Jeff, know what was going on, but it was necessary. Just as I had predicted, he immediately thought the worst. Or at least he appeared this way to me. He confronted me and said, "Twirp (my nickname), I am going to bring you to the hospital, and everywhere else you may need to go." He needed to be involved in my process. It was difficult to look at his face that so much resembles my mother, without being reminded of her. His six foot two inch frame suddenly looked like a small child's.

"Jeff," I said, "I love you very much, but you have a wife and children and I have a husband and children. I appreciate the attention, but you must allow Michael to take care of me." This was like trying to drive a nail into granite. He was not going to give. So I compromised, with the permission of Michael, "Jeff, I thought maybe you could pick me up from the hospital so that Michael could be home when the girls come home, and my dear friend Andrea will drop me off so that we can pray together on the way up." It worked. He thought he had won. I suppose over the years I have acquired a talent for working all the Phelan men the right way!

I managed to get through all of the pre-admission tests and set my sights for Friday, surgery day. I decided to carry my Saint Christopher medallion in my hand to the hospital for reassurance. Although I don't normally wear much jewelry, I was in the habit of wearing a gold rope chain with the medallion because it was a special gift from my brother, Jeff. Coming home I realized that I didn't have the medallion on today. I looked everywhere and I couldn't find it. Panic set in. I thought, "Oh my God, this is a jinx. Something terrible is about to happen."

I tried to collect myself and realized just how ridiculous I was being, but my insecurities were still getting the best of me. Everything was racing through my mind so fast that I couldn't understand what was really happening. It all seemed so much larger than life that even the smallest negative incident was enough to make me panic. I insisted on finding the medallion, and made myself nuts looking for two days. Finally, my brother Jeff decided to give me his chain and medallion for my peace of mind. Ironically, I would not be permitted to wear any jewelry during the surgery, so what difference did it make?

That night it hit me. Just what kind of power did I think this medallion possessed? My faith was not a material thing. I was just feeling so terribly vulnerable, and thought that somehow it could offer me some peace.

I prayed that my realization be acknowledged. My faith was in something much greater, and this held the peace I was seeking. It was OK if I didn't have the silly medallion. I didn't need it.

I got up in the morning and went downstairs to do some laundry. Beside the washing machine were several empty water bottles. I moved them out of my way and couldn't believe what I saw. My chain and medallion were sitting at the bottom of one of the bottles! How on earth could they have gotten in there? The mouth of the bottle itself was only about two inches in diameter. It all began to make some sense. It wasn't until I realized where my faith really was that the medallion came back to me.

I began to meditate and do visualization, sending positive affirmations to my cells. But, something was just not right. I kept getting the feeling that the lump in my left breast was compromising my health in a way I dreaded. I had no feelings in the right breast. I began to feel very inferior to the powers around me, wondering if I could possibly affect the outcome of this situation. In fact, I was beginning to doubt my own strength. How could this have happened? I believed that nothing or no one could make me feel unimportant or inferior unless I consented to it. I wanted to matter. I promised myself to claim my own power, and that no matter what the outcome might be I would stand strong. My path might appear obstructed in many ways, but no rocks, mountains or streams would keep me from walking it.

I vowed to always love and honor my*self*, as I had done with others. This was especially difficult since I believed in my heart that I had a part in the making of this illness, and had possibly even nurtured it in some ways. How could I love myself knowing this? It was difficult but ever so necessary to fulfill this promise in order to go on. Yes, one of the hardest lessons in one's life was to learn to love oneself.

Friday. Of course I was nervous, but nobody would be able to tell. Andrea arrived, and she agreed to let me drive. I desperately needed that little bit of control! She comforted me by promising to pray for me, and that everything would be fine. It was the next best thing to having my own mother with me. The warmth and love Andrea generated seemed endless. The nurses were wonderful and I was immediately brought back to change into a gown. I had intentionally worn my favorite thick cotton socks and planned to leave them on, convinced that if my feet were cold I would be very unhappy. A nurse took one look at them and laughed out loud. I felt like a complete idiot.

She said, "Gee, I have had a lot of experiences, but never was anyone so insistent on wearing a special pair of socks. I can only conclude that they are special and since you already warned us that you get bitchy when your feet are cold, I suppose we'll humor you!"

There was always a nurse around. Dr. Herman was in surgery, and I was next. A very attractive male nurse anesthetist came in to insert the IV needle into my hand. Actually, it felt more like it was driving up my arm. He asked, "Are you all right?" while batting his beautiful brown eyes. I was so embarrassed. He must have noticed all the sweat pouring off my forehead. He continued, "I can give you something just to relax you. Dr. Herman informed me that you're here for just a local procedure, but recommended that I have something on hand since he will biopsy two spots, not just one." As he went on the idea of *feeling good* was beginning to make a drug sound pretty appealing.

Dr. Herman was next door and I could hear him speaking to an older woman. He said, "I have good news. We are certain that the small mass we removed was benign and I don't want you to worry about a thing." I thought, YES! He was on a roll today. I will be hearing those same words very shortly. I tried to ignore a persistent inner voice, preparing me for the worst. Dr. Herman peeked his head around my curtain. He was dressed in scrubs so I couldn't see the attractive bald spot on the top of his head or rub it for good luck!

He explained, "I am going to make two incisions starting with the left side. It should not take very long and you will be allowed to leave shortly after we are through. I am really looking forward to sitting down with you and hearing more about your MLD work. Maybe we can incorporate it into my office somehow?"

How can I ever forget that good looking male nurse sitting directly above me while they were strapping my arms up and exposing my 34 C's for all to see? Sure, he sees them all day, but these were mine. This was different! There was a bit of a sting and then the nurse juiced me up with something that would have made even the most miserable person happy.

I couldn't just lie there like a dummy, so I decided to strike up some conversation with Mr. Handsome. I asked him if he had any children. He replied, yes, one daughter—two years old. For some strange reason I was relieved. I must have thought that since he was probably married, my breasts wouldn't mean all that much to him. Then, all of a sudden (and I blame this on the drug), the most bizarre, yet hysterical story popped into my head about Meg.

I let it pour out. "One Saturday, I had come home from work to find Meg up in a tree with a skirt on. I suppose she has trouble with which side was going to dominate her, the feminine side or the tomboy side. So she just mixed them, and sometimes, not well! After giving Mike a five-minute lecture about letting his daughter climb trees in a skirt, I yelled to Meg to get down and put some pants on. On that note she did just that. She *slid* all the way down in her skirt. All I could say was, "*Ouch!*" She didn't show any emotion.

I followed after about five minutes and found her sitting on the bathroom toilet, stripped from the waist down, with her head between her legs. She had some little scratches from sliding down, but nothing to get alarmed about. I told her to wash up and get dressed. Just as I turned to leave she belted out a scream that the entire neighborhood must have heard. She began sobbing hysterically. Mike ran in, followed by Cara, and our dog, Kai. We all looked at Meg in the same pitiful way and asked her what on earth the matter was.

She replied, "I got a hole in my bum from sliding down the tree," referring to her vagina of course. Well Mike nearly wet himself and had to leave the room. Cara stuck around to see what approach I was going to take on this one. At first, I wanted to tell her that this was the same hole she stuffed gummy bears up two years earlier, but I knew that wouldn't go anywhere. It took about 20 minutes of unprepared lecturing to convince her that it indeed belonged to her as a part of her "girl" body. This, of course, involved using pictures. After all, she wasn't going to take my word for it. So, now boys have a penis (which she thought was appalling!) and girls have vaginas.

We were just about through convincing when Cara began to wish she had exited with her father. Meg looked up at Cara and begged, "Can I see yours?" Well of course, mother stuck around to watch this! I still can't remember how she got out of it, but she did."

So here was this poor guy listening to my pathetic attempt to converse from the surgery table. I realized when I stopped talking that the entire room fell silent. At that moment a valve opened in me and my emotions flooded out. I cried so hard it was impossible to stop. Since I couldn't move my arms, the nurse had to keep wiping my tears. I knew something had to be wrong. I kept praying that it would soon be over, and finally, it was.

I was wheeled out into a recovery area. The medication wore off rapidly and all I wanted to do was go home. I kept asking the nurse why I was crying so much. There was no sign of Dr. Herman. I just remembered that Jeff would be waiting for me and I wanted to make sure I didn't look like I'd been crying. If he noticed my face being red, I thought I would tell him it was because they had wrapped this incredibly tight corset around my chest to stop the bleeding, and the blood was being pushed up into my head. Pretty good thinking, huh?

Before I knew it, Jeff had talked his way into the recovery area. A few flashes of those green eyes can get him in anywhere. He appeared so solemn and concerned. I said, "I'm ready to go, but I have to wait for Dr. Herman." Oh my God. Dr. Herman. I prayed so fast that he wouldn't give me any bad news in front of Jeff. At that moment he walked towards me and I had to find the strength not to cry. I knew the look on his face was not the look I had been hoping to see.

Dr. Herman sat down on the other side of me, "Linda, the tissue is going to require further biopsy before we know exactly what we are looking at." I felt both frustrated and relieved—frustrated, that he didn't just go ahead and say "malignant" when he must have known the truth. But, I was also relieved that he didn't say this in front of Jeff. I agreed to come in the following Friday when he would have the pathology report.

Jeff took me home in silence. I tried to make light conversation, with no success. It was pouring rain and I said that there was an old wives' tale that rain was good luck.

With that he replied, "I hope we have a damn flood."

"Be courageous, enduring, vigilant and above all, be sincere, with perfect honesty. Then you will be able to face all difficulties."

—The Mother
Pondicherry , India

CHAPTER 3

THE DIAGNOSIS

Mike was happy to see me safe. Later that night, I tried to explain my experience in the operating room but he didn't want any part of it. I was worried for him but also terribly hurt. This was a time when I really needed him, yet he was so far away. I had to be strong without him.

The week was filled with anticipation and fear. I kept thinking my left breast was cancerous. Twenty-nine years old with breast cancer. My dentist friend, Paul, was my last patient on Friday. He's a very nice man with a mild disposition, and very easy to talk to.

"Linda," he offered, "Kay and I don't have any plans tonight, so why don't you let me come with you to Providence. You know, just someone to talk to and keep you company." It was not until that moment that I realized Mike never even offered to be with me tonight. Friends, family and even patients were worried and offering their support and company, and my husband was sitting at home waiting for me to walk in the door with good news.

The phone rang just before I left the office and it was Michael, "Why don't we go to dinner tonight and celebrate, once this is all over and behind us?" I thought, my God, he's in trouble. I didn't agree to dinner, but I did tell him I would phone him before I left Dr. Herman's office. I turned down Paul's offer, several times telling him that I was better off alone. Intuitively I knew by the time I got home I would have several calls to make: Steve (my chiropractor), his wife, my friend Lyn, Deb, Rosemary, Kevin, Rosie and probably others.

I had not even phoned my Aunt Marge in California to inform her of the biopsies. I knew she'd be shocked, and I couldn't justify doing that to her until I knew something certain. The drive seemed to take an eternity. Once there, I waited for what felt like hours. My hands were like ice cubes. I didn't have the same great feeling entering the office that I had experienced the first time.

Dr. Herman entered the room, staring down at a piece of paper. I thought, take a deep breath Linda and, whatever you do, contain yourself. He looked up at me. I thought, this poor man...what a nasty job. He must dread these moments. He said, "Linda, sometimes the least expected outcome turns out to be true."

I gasped. I knew all along, and yet the reality of hearing a physician confirm it was shocking. I was in some dark, echoing tunnel when I heard the word *breasts*. Not singular, but plural. Rudely, I interrupted him, "What about the right breast?" He suddenly realized that I hadn't heard a word he had said. I had bilateral breast cancer.

"Both?"

"Yes."

My God. I struggled to regain my composure, although I'm sure that my borderline hysteria was very noticeable. I began sizing him up, wondering if I could deck him. I thought, well, he is about my height, light build, gee whiz Linda what are you thinking?!

He went on..."The pathologist could not quite classify the tumors, but agreed that they best resembled what is known as Medullary Breast Carcinoma. But, it usually only occurs in one breast and one site and here both of your breasts are involved." Of course, I had to be unusual. He continued, "This particular kind of breast cancer only makes up for about 2 percent of all breast cancers. It has a fair to good prognosis if treated early."

I looked him square in the eyes, "Look, I want the breasts OFF ASAP!!"

"Linda, think about it. Even get a second opinion if it will make you feel better, but I think we must sit down with a multidisciplinary group before any final decisions are made." But, I knew I wanted and would have the damn things *off*.

Dr. Herman added, "There is another procedure that has become quite popular. I can do a re-incision of the tumor site to make sure it is all cleaned out and dissect the lymph nodes to check for possible metastases (spreading of the tumor) and follow up with radiation."

"I want them off."

"The statistics reveal that the prognosis is just as favorable."

None of this even mattered to me. Somewhere along the line, I must have subconsciously made the decision to have both breasts removed if the disease ever invaded me. It was not a question of conserving, or aesthetics, but rather a question of what was best for me. I needed this to regain my sanity. I felt as though I had completely left the planet.

The doctor continued, "Let's make another appointment for all of us to meet, including your husband." My husband, oh yeah, I thought, that fool sitting at home waiting to go to dinner.

"I will make you a copy of the pathology report before you leave, and I want you to know that I am available any time, day or night, for you or your husband." That was very nice, and I didn't dare embarrass myself by telling him that my husband was home shaving, waiting to go out to dinner.

Pat gave me an appointment for the following Monday to meet with the multidisciplinary group. She was at a loss for words, so we just exchanged smiles. I asked her if she could telephone my husband and just let him know that I was on my way. "Sure Linda, is there anything else I can do?"

"Yes, could you please tell me that this is all a bad dream, and I will wake in the morning to singing birds and the wind?"

Dr. Herman came back up front, "Linda I am going to go ahead and reserve the operating room since I know that you are very anxious and I feel the sooner we get going the better."

I barely made it to the car and collapsed into a screaming fit. I had a million questions. What am I doing? What do I know? What am I learning? Am I so far off center in life, that I will never come back? I felt alienated from the entire universe, rejected from my sphere due to imperfections. I held my eyes tightly together, waiting for the whole thing to disappear. But, it didn't.

Somehow, some way, some time ago, I must have decided to live this experience as part of my learning or healing. I knew I needed to embrace it openheartedly, in order to suck up all it had to offer me. Yet I was terrified. It was dark out by the time I left the parking area. I had no conception of time, no idea just how long I had been sitting there with my eyes closed. Before I knew it, I found myself pulling off the highway. Subconsciously, I knew I needed someone right at that very moment.

I found myself driving to the store where Andrea worked, with only a vague idea of where it was located. It felt like my guardian angel directed my car right into a parking space just outside the store. I went in and panicked when I didn't see Andrea. I must have looked wild because the other people in there responded with a look of fear in their eyes. I blurted out Andrea's name, and a woman said she would get her from the ladies room.

I waited outside, wondering why I came here. Somehow, I was compelled by my emotions. I was afraid that Andrea wouldn't be able to handle what I was about to tell her, and I would just die if there were two loonies blubbering in the store.

Andrea came out and studied my face. Feeling the hysteria in the air, she approached me, cool as a cucumber. I told her I had cancer. I will never forget how composed she was, even as those words were leaving my lips—no sign of shock or upset. She knew what she had to do for me, and she was doing it very well.

Andrea put her own emotions on hold so that she could deal with me. She stood in front of me and took my hand, "All right, Linda. You have been through quite a lot in your short twenty-nine years of life, and you have grown stronger in many ways through each experience. This, too, you will grow from. With my help and prayers, and the help of many others who will be sent to you, you will be OK."

I thought to myself, who was this person? This was not the Andrea that I knew, but I supposed it was the inner Andrea that I loved. It never even dawned on me that her mother had died from this very disease. She promised that she and Joe would pray for me. I swore silently that I would never again doubt her strength. She provided an emotional fulcrum that allowed me to rebalance.

On my way home, I talked to God—as I did routinely while driving. I asked Him, "If I needed a message, why couldn't I have just fallen down some stairs and broken a few bones?"

God said to me, "You have already had broken bones, so that experience is used up."

"What about an accident, like a car accident?"

"Well, that too has been used."

"You mean to tell me that it's going to take an experience of such great impact to direct me back to my path?" I supposed this was it. Breast cancer was to be my next path. I wondered, if I conquer this one, what do I get? Maybe some sort of a trophy, or even a victory plaque. Or better yet, a nice uneventful, sometimes boringly simple life? I believed that if I stayed centered and on my path, I could live this kind of simple and loving life. Why did it seem so difficult?

I never questioned my paths before this. I believe that long before we come to earth, we choose the paths which are necessary for our spiritual growth. So far, my paths have always taken me to the light of higher places. I decided I must again have faith that this experience would lead me to greater spiritual growth. The challenge is always to remain true to your faith even when you don't yet understand the message that is being brought to you. If one can't trust their faith, they will spend an eternity in doubt.

Driving home was just a blur. I pulled into the driveway and wondered what Mike and the girls were doing. I was not at all sure how I was going to present this to them, but I trusted my instincts to handle it correctly. Boy, was I wrong. I barely made it in the door and halfway up the foyer before Mike appeared with shaving cream on his face. He was actually getting ready to go to dinner! For a few seconds, I stood frozen in disbelief. I thought, "That bastard, how could he?" I could feel the anger building inside me.

I shouted at him, "I have breast cancer, OK? And not just in one breast but *both! How* does that sound? Can you believe it?" I must have sounded like a crazed lunatic. He grabbed me so fast that I thought he might kill me with the razor in his hands. No more denial. Reality hit with a million pounds of impact. I rambled on for about ten minutes, repeating every word that Dr. Herman had said. I showed Mike the books, movies and cassettes he had given me to listen to. I told him that if he felt the need, he could phone the doctor for information or reassurance.

Slowly, Mike and I pulled apart until we were finally arms length and looked into the deepest, most soulful part of our eyes. At that moment, I knew that Mike would be everything to me in the coming months. We agreed that once I got washed up, we would sit and talk and listen. He said there were several phone calls while I was gone. I guess I expected them. I didn't know if I should wait until morning, or phone them now.

I looked at the list: Deb, Jeff, Kevin, Lyn, Steve, and my dear friend Beth. I knew I couldn't put it off until morning, so I made the first call to Deb. What could she say? I tried so hard to hold back the tears and emotion, but was only partially successful. Mike thought I was torturing myself by calling and going through this. I told her that I was scared. "The word *cancer* is such a terrible word. I mean, why would they use a word for such a terrible disease that has been borrowed from the Latin word meaning crabs? I would much prefer a bad case of crabs any day, over this."

"Me too," Deb added. We had to chuckle a little. I hung up and phoned Lyn. She was strong and supportive. She would let Steve know what was going on, and they would be in touch. Kevin was silent. By now I had begun to build up strength. I thanked God for telling me to make these phone calls. The more I spoke about it, the deeper it sunk in. It was no longer an illusion, but rather a bold reality. I couldn't keep Kevin on the phone because I knew he was uncomfortable. Here was a reputable, successful attorney, not knowing what to say. It was almost funny in a way. He was the exact opposite of what people consider normal for an attorney. He was a big teddy bear with an equally big heart.

My sister, Rosemary, was next. She answered the phone, and I said, "Ro, I have cancer." I think she went into a state of shock because I didn't hear a word for about ten minutes. For her and my brother Jeff, this news brought up many unresolved feelings about my mothers illness, making it even more difficult to handle. I told her I would keep her posted as to what I chose to do and when I would be doing it. I couldn't bring myself to call Jeff. I knew I would have to handle my approach to him a bit differently and I needed to give the whole thing some serious thought.

I was equally concerned for my daughters. Fortunately, Meg was totally unaware of the seriousness of the ongoing discussions. Cara, on the other hand, was fully aware and tried her best not to look too alarmed. As I experienced my illness, I never tried to keep my voice down or hide what was being said. Most of the time, I was totally unaware that she was even around, even though she was visible. It somehow didn't matter. I think this was for the best. Cara and I have always lived and shared our lives in a very open and understanding way, and this was no time to change.

This experience was real and she needed to see my emotions, the ones I longed to see from my mother. I gave her a question-and-answer book. I told her that my cancer was being caught at an early stage, and that I would do all I needed to do to be well again. I only needed her support, her love and her patience. What she may or may not have learned about disease, or breast cancer, was not comparable to my situation. We were all individuals.

Cara was so confused. She had always had this terrific image of her young, healthy mother. Why should this be happening? It really made no sense to her. I had to be very careful in choosing my words so that I wouldn't plant the same destructive seeds of fear in her. I truly believed that she had nothing to worry about since she was really still a child. I knew that my experience, and how I encountered it and presented it to her, would have great impact on her development. I would show her how our intention, intuition and will can turn the most devastating of situations into a time of joy.

I realized that every word, hug and howl we exchanged over the next year would mean a great deal. We would engage in many loving discussions about life and enlightenment, and she would always have the choice to speak to a professional if she decided. I believed our connection was a strong one, and we would be all right.

Lastly, I phoned my dearest friend, Beth, who lived in Martha's Vineyard. Since we first met in massage therapy school, we had been very close. People thought we were sisters. We had about the same build, with blue eyes and the same small Irish-looking face. I had never heard anything negative or harsh come out of her mouth. Beth expressed herself in such a lovely way, as only she could. Married recently, both she and her husband, Steve, were triathletes and seemed to be in constant training for one event or another. After our talk, she assured me we would see each other very soon.

I knew that it was now time for Mike and me to sit down and talk. I had a long road ahead of me, and some very important choices to make. It was to be a long night.

*"In search of my lost innocence, I walked out a door. At the time I
believed I was looking for a purpose, but I found instead, the meaning
of choice."*

—Liv Ullman

All night long I felt like my physical body was all that existed. My
mind seemed so far away, like in a dream, a frightening dream. I couldn't
feel or think much of anything. Mike and I watched the video first. I
despised it. Nothing they had to say interested me. There were three
women, the youngest was 46 years old. None of them were in similar
situations. As for the cassette tape, well, it was lucky to still be intact. I put
it in and listened to three older woman tell their heart wrenching stories
about cancer, and their "why me's." Why me? Why me? *Aagh! I* could not
tolerate whining. The books were OK, but just OK. Finally, in despair, I
said to Mike, "Why don't we take a trip to the Brown University library
and try deciphering my pathology so that I have an idea of what is going
on inside my body?"

"I think that is a terrific idea and it will make us both feel like we are
doing something about it." I needed to go into my office and clear up
some paperwork, so we could leave. I wanted to go to the bookstore and
buy every book pertaining to breast cancer. Yet in my heart I knew that
this was a time in my life when courage rather than knowledge was what
I needed to continue on my path. All night long I felt like someone was
sitting inside of my head and stirring my mind with a mixer. I was sure of
myself in one sense—I knew I would remain strong—yet at the same time
I was terribly confused. It was so simple, I had cancer, but reality was also
the fact that it was everything but simple. Even with that in mind I decided I would try to stick to the simple.

"Whatever is the difficulty, if we keep truly quiet the solution will come."

—The Mother
Pondicherry, India

The birds were sitting outside our window in the bird-feeder when we awakened. I had only had a few hours sleep, but I woke feeling totally refreshed and energized. I looked out at the dynamic autumn day that greeted me and was filled with a grand essence of life. I spoke to Mike quietly, "You know, it's like my leaves are falling because it is time for transition, but they will come back dancing, and joyful, overflowing with health and vitality."

I was sure that people chose their soulmates for many reasons. I had always felt that Mike loved my impulsive, philosophical ways. They were deep within him, too, but difficult for him to let out. I justified this for him. I said philosophy was a definite topic of curiosity for me, but if you were not careful, it could pull the cloud out from under the angel.

He just laughed, "Honey, I want to see your leaves come back dancing too."

I phoned my guardian angel, Karen, knowing that she would be home from her trip. There was much to fill her in on. "Do you have a copy of your pathology?" she asked me. I read her my pathology report and when I finished, there was a slight pause. She said, "Linda, would you mind if I brought you up to Boston to see my surgeon, who is also a close friend of mine, to get a second opinion?"

"Karen, you just read my mind, but why doesn't that surprise me? I would really like the pathologist there to read my slides and see if he agrees with the original report."

"Good idea. Call the hospital and let them know that you will be picking up your slides at eight-thirty, Monday morning. I will bring some nursing books of mine that will tell you a little about that particular kind of breast cancer." I was so grateful. Why was she doing this for me? She said, "I'll call ahead to my doctors office and let him know that he'll have to squeeze you in Monday."

Karen had been a nurse practitioner for several years and, in the middle of chemotherapy, decided to open her own real estate business. I liked her attitude and spunk, and of course, agreed with everything she said. I left for my office in the morning as Mike and I had agreed. It was nearly impossible for me to focus on paper work so I walked next door to give Kay and Paul the results I had promised. They were shocked. I left them a copy of the pathology report to see if anything sounded familiar to them.

I had totally forgotten about Jeff, when all of a sudden he walked through my door, "I called your house and Mike said you were here. Why didn't you call me back last night?" I could see the hurt in his face and the darkness in his eyes. I also knew that he must have assumed the worst. I didn't do him any favors by not calling him. There was no time to compose a script for the ideal response, although I certainly would have appreciated one. I told him that the biopsies were malignant. I went on to tell him that we felt the cancer was caught early and I was going to do everything humanly possible to recover fully. I would recover from this. Like me, he never got past the word *cancer*. Damn that word. I wanted so badly to hug him and tell him that I was not Mom. It would be different with me, but he left before I could see him cry.

I fell to my knees in tears praying to God that there would be a good purpose for putting everybody I loved through such pain. I could manage, but I wanted everybody else to survive it too. I felt it was my job. It would change their lives forever, especially two that were of most concern to me now. The first was Jeff. Many positive things could come from this for him as long as he chose to utilize it in a good way. This experience could resolve the negative feelings he stored away for many years about cancer. They were his innermost feelings that came from watching my mother be taken by the same disease. He would see me get well again, and value life and loving more than he could have ever imagined.

My second concern was for Mike, my soulmate. The man I married who swears he had no faith in any one God or creator. I would bring witness to him, and by the end of this experience, he would believe. He would open that pained childhood heart of his to light and love, and lo and behold, never be the same! Before me, I had the opportunity to change and touch many lives in the most positive, enlightening way.

When we finally made it to the library, Mike said, "I'm so sorry that I couldn't put Jeff off, but he was desperate to see you."

"That's all right, honey. I knew it would be difficult. I have a strong feeling that it will all work out."

We flooded our heads with rivers of information on cancer. It always seems much more serious when reading about it in medical books. Not that cancer isn't serious, it is about as serious as it gets. But, when you think about the disease, in reality it comes down to a bunch of stupid cells. Literally stupid. They are cells that are dividing without control of their growth, and yes, they eventually can cluster together and form a life-threatening mass.

Then I read on. I had the so-called worst family scenario: both my mother and her sister died from breast cancer. So my cells inherited the genetic imprint of how to be stupid and create a problem. Scientists think that it is a combination of factors that create cells which have lost control of their growth. These factors can be things like genetics, ultraviolet radiation, chemicals and pollutants. And I would add *negative energy* to the list.

Since there are two copies of every gene in a cell, it can take two errors in the cell's growth control to create a cancer cell. This means that my genetics gives me one factor, and I must live very carefully to avoid getting another factor.

Now it was important for me to stop feeding my cells with negative energy from my thoughts, and retrain the messages my cells were receiving. Many people, from gurus in India to American doctors, have shown that your state of mind directly affects your health. One simple explanation for this related the state of your energy—positive or negative—to your immune system. People who were happy and positive had a stronger immune system which could fight off disease.

For me, negative energy came from the emotions I had repressed since my Mother's death. Since childhood, I kept fear, anger and sadness deep in my heart surrounding the issue of mothering. As a result, all my decisions about mothering my own daughters were colored by my need to make up for what I missed. My daughters would be *over* mothered, over controlled because of my need to be the perfect mother. To overcome my negative energy and heal my cells, I needed to look deeply within myself. I had to confront the feelings and responses I denied for so long. Sounds so easy doesn't it...easier said than done.

The challenge began. Now I had the opportunity to test my mental, spiritual and physical self and begin living my life focused on health. I was fully aware that if I didn't meet this challenge, it would come back to me. In some ways I would be reliving my mother's life.

We read all our minds could digest, and then some. We spent over one hundred dollars on books...cancer and vitamin books, visualization books, breast cancer books, centering and meditation books (things which I already practiced regularly), and a few other books as Christmas presents. I loved the Christmas season so much that I tried to have my shopping done early so I could enjoy the month of December even more. The spirit was strong and everything felt so magical, the nearer the much celebrated day came.

CHAPTER 4

LISTENING FOR THE ANSWERS

Monday morning, eight o'clock, and Karen was in the driveway. I told Mike that I would meet him at the hospital by five p.m. He held me so close to him that I thought he was never going to let me go. From there, we would meet with Dr. Herman and Dr. Gabrielle Masko, a radiation oncologist. Karen and I finally got our chance to meet face-to-face. I poured out my endless thanks for her generous support and time. She was happy to be there for me, like any angel. I thought it was healing for her to be helping me.

We picked up the slides and proceeded to Boston. She had arranged for the slides to be brought over to The Deaconess, and for me to be checked out by her surgeon, Dr. Barton. It was the strangest feeling, sitting there with a little box containing the actual cells from my own body. Cells that were threatening my life. The biggest thing Karen and I had in common was breast cancer. Karen broke the tension, "You know, you're going to beat this shitty disease, don't you?"

"I'm going to do my best, but I'm terrified."

"Well let it rip, Linda, because the more you hold it in, the more damage it can do to you."

"I have no time to let it rip. I have so much to think about, I have to stay in control. It's just not the right time yet."

We arrived in what seemed like no time at all. The slides were immediately taken over next door and we waited to see Dr. Barton. He was in emergency surgery and it was uncertain how long he would be. Karen said, with her eyes dancing, "I know. We'll go over to the Chestnut Hill Mall. And then to lunch! We'll put some pleasure into this day." That we did. We had lunch at Legal Seafood and went back to his office.

They took me immediately. Karen made the introduction. I felt like I was sitting in the principle's office. Dr. Barton was a large white-haired man, obviously very serious about his work. There were no smiles exchanged, just a let's-get-down-to-business look.

"Tell me about your family history." I did. He said, "Tell me about your sex life, do you achieve orgasm?" I had to ask him to repeat the question. Orgasm? What the hell does that have to do with anything? Oh well...I answered of course. He discussed *everything*! He examined me from head to toe and we met back in his office where Karen was waiting for me.

I sat down and Dr. Barton said, "OK, here is my opinion. You are an otherwise healthy twenty-nine-year-old woman with an ominous family history of breast cancer. You have bilateral breast cancer yourself. My recommendation is a bilateral, modified mastectomy followed by aggressive chemotherapy and, quite possibly, radiation." Someone knocked on the door. It was his nurse. She handed him a copy of the second opinion pathology, and it confirmed the original. I did not have a *typical* cancer. Leave it to me to have something different. I was blown into another solar system. Karen reached for my hand, but I knew the contact would push all the buttons for my emotions to flow. I was not comfortable with that happening right then.

I felt somehow annoyed with this doctor. Then I realized that I was really needy and confused, hoping he would give me some consolation. But, I had to face facts. I was here for a second opinion and that was what this man was honestly giving me. It wasn't his fault that his opinion supported the bad news I'd already heard. I thanked him and we went on our way home. By now, my head was splitting, and we were running very late. I telephoned Michael from my angel's car phone and said I'd be late.

He understood, "OK, but how are you?" I asked if we could discuss it later. Karen dropped me off with very few words exchanged. But, she made it clear that I could call her anytime I needed to. I told her I couldn't thank her enough. She reminded me that's what friends are for.

Poor Mike received the short, fast version of the day, before we met with Dr. Strair. She walked into the room and I instantly felt relieved. First, I suppose because she was a woman, and second, because she was very close to my own age.

"I must apologize. I have not had time to obtain a copy of your pathology report."

"Quite all right, we have it memorized!" Then I began reciting it all to her and what I couldn't remember, Mike did.

Dr. Strair was amused and then began, "Another surgery is necessary. Whether you have a re-incision on the left or not, is up to you but I do recommend a mastectomy on the right due to the size of the tumor and it's deep margins. I am going to reserve any recommendations on the chemotherapy. I need to see the lymph node pathology before I can make a recommendation. I would probably recommend CMF which seems to be the standard drugs of choice for breast cancer if all of your nodes are negative for cancer, which stands for cytoxin, methotrexate, and 5 FU. The side effects from these are minimal nausea, and possibly some hair loss, but not necessarily. This would be used if all the lymph nodes came back negative for cancer."

Dr. Strair continued, "If you have any positive nodes, my recommendation will be CAF, cytoxan, adriamycin, and 5 FU. The side effects would be the less desirable with a 99% chance of losing all your hair, and possible severe nausea. They have some drugs they use to help with the nausea, but it is a matter of finding which one would work the best, which is, of course, a trial and error thing."

Oh my. By now, the only hope to hang onto was not to have any positive nodes. Regardless of any of the recommendations, these were all choices which had to be made by me and only me. People expressed their opinions if I asked, but every decision was mine. Dr. Strair said that Dr. Masko could better help me with the decision about whether to have the re-incision or the modified mastectomies. What I didn't tell her was that I had already decided to have the mastectomies. It was helpful to hear from a female medical standpoint that this was the favorable choice. It seemed that we only asked for advice when we already knew all the answers. We just wished we didn't. We thanked her and proceeded to Dr. Herman's office.

I could barely stand up on my two feet by this point. Just when I felt at my weakest, sitting in the exam room waiting for Dr. Masko, I closed my eyes for a few seconds and I heard my guardian angel saying to me, "It's all right, don't be afraid. Don't worry, I am here." I opened my eyes and there stood Dr. Masko. I must have had my eyes closed when she entered the room and she was respecting my moment of meditation.

Dr. Masko was a very beautiful woman, with very reassuring eyes, and, *yikes*, very cold hands! She reviewed my biopsy report and said, in her opinion, I had very little choice but to have the modified mastectomy on the right breast because of the size of the tumor and its possible permeation. As for the left, it was a candidate for re-incision with possible radiation therapy. Then I asked the infamous question, "What would you do if you were me?" Of course, this was a very selfish question to ask, but I felt in the selfish mood. She didn't respond immediately, which made me realize that I had just done something pretty stupid.

I apologized, "I'm sorry for putting you on the spot like that. The fact is, I have already made my decision. I want both breasts removed."

She looked into my eyes and smiled, "I completely agree with your decision Linda. It is a tough one and I can only admire you for making it." I was so elated that another professional agreed with me. Karen did also, but I wasn't counting her (no offense Karen). I knew in my heart it didn't matter what anyone else would choose, because what was best for them, might not be best for me. The one thing I was sure of was that we all had the freedom to choose and make appropriate choices for ourselves.

I met with Dr. Herman. Mike joined us and together we discussed the future of my diseased breasts. Dr. Herman looked at me and said with great respect that he realized from the moment I informed him of my choice, that I knew what I needed to do. He was so happy that I was comfortable with the decision. He looked at Mike and then me, and asked, "Are you interested in reconstruction?"

"Well I haven't given it much thought. I certainly do not want to go through several operations, so if I were to say 'yes,' could it be done at the same time?" I looked at Mike as he said that he didn't want me going through any unnecessary surgery.

Then he added what I needed to hear, "You don't need to have any of that to please me." But, I don't think he was thinking about all those wonderful nights, in our future, of dancing in Aruba (he hated dancing, but there was still hope!) And me doing cartwheels on the sandy beach with the girls. I could deal with one prosthesis falling out, but if both my boobs fell out at the same time, I wouldn't be a happy camper!

It really was a choice of convenience as well as esthetics. I was so active, and planned on remaining so. I wanted those two bumps in my braless dresses. And besides, I despised bras. Cosmetic surgery would give me the choice of wearing one or not. Then I made the decision to have reconstruction. Dr. Herman explained the normal procedure for this and we found out that it would require additional surgery. If I were having the flap surgery, where they take excess fat from the abdomen, it could be done at the same time. But, I didn't have nearly enough extra for even one boob, let alone two.

The silicone prostheses were inserted under the pectoral muscle on the chest, but before they could put them in, they have to insert what was known as expander bags which they inflated over a three-month period until the desired size was achieved, at which time, the permanent prosthesis could then be inserted. To have them inserted immediately was usually impossible. It would be like going from normal to eight months pregnant, without allowing time for the tissue to expand.

I reminded him that the only way I would have reconstruction, was if I could have it during the original surgery. I even had some volunteers to donate some of their excess fatty tissue if need be!

"Discuss it with Dr. Barrall, Linda, since I cannot speak for him. Dr. Barrall is who I would refer you to. I think you will like him and I can tell you quite honestly that he does beautiful work." Well, how beautiful can two bags of silicone stuffed under a muscle be, I wondered? Yet, it did please me to hear that Dr. Herman had such high regard for the man as a surgeon. Dr. Herman asked, "Would you like me to call him?"

Mike and I just looked at each other, "Isn't it a bit late?"

"No problem, this is important...I'll call him at home." Once he had Dr. Barrall on the phone, he briefed him on my case and said that the operating room was reserved for a week from Wednesday. This was the first I had heard anything this concrete. Mike and I looked at each other with a sick sense of excitement. We wanted all of this behind us.

Dr. Barrall agreed to meet with me to discuss reconstruction, but he would not be available to do any surgery on the reserved date. This was the day he saw patients in his office—a very busy day. I wanted to cry. Everything seemed to be going right along. Dr. Herman suggested I phone him in the morning to get an appointment as soon as possible and discuss it with him. I wondered what was the use if he couldn't do the surgery. I just wouldn't have it done. This was wrong, because I knew I wanted it done. I just felt that if we were talking about *my* body, then I would have it done *my* way!

I was scheduled for pre-admissions tests on Wednesday. These would include blood work and a special test to make sure my liver functions were normal. This was just a preliminary work-up to make certain there was no metastases in my liver. Also, a chest x-ray, for the same reason. The thought of having these tests horrified me. It never occurred to me that the cancer could have gone somewhere other than the breast, yet I was certain it hadn't.

The most frightening test I was scheduled for was a bone scan, to be done on Saturday. I would be injected with a radioactive dye, and sent away for three hours. Then I'd return and be scanned by a gamma ray machine which would light up any abnormalities. When we parted with Dr. Herman, I knew that I probably wouldn't see him until the day of surgery. I thanked him from the bottom of my heart for being there. He smiled and hugged me. I knew I was being well taken care of.

Mike and I agreed that we would tag our Christmas tree at Little Compton Tree Farm the day of my bone scan. He knew I was terrified. Since tagging our tree was one of my favorite things to do, it might make the day easier. Trying to prepare myself, Cara and Meg for what was coming was difficult. I spoke to Jeff and he seemed to have taken a turn. Although it seems to involve a bit of rebellion, he was going to make damn sure that I got well! He insisted on being the designated chemotherapy driver, and doing anything else that was needed. If it weren't so serious it would have been comical. I told him that no decisions had been made yet about chemotherapy but he would be the first to know.

I had to be firm in letting him know that Mike really needed to be with me if I chose that route. But, if we needed him, we would certainly call him. I knew that doing this for me would just be a heart wrenching way to relive the terrible memories of my mother's chemotherapy. He had gone with her and witnessed the terrible reactions firsthand.

I would not allow my children to see me physically ill, if I decided to go that route. That was the only event I refused for them to witness. It would take some creative planning on Mike's part, but it would be done. I would hide nothing else. My daughters would play an active role in my recovery, which I hoped would give them a sense of involvement rather than alienation.

Deb and I spent some time together discussing office issues, and she was confident that everything at the office would be fine. Not the same without me, she admitted, but she could handle any possible problems that might arise. I was so blessed to have such wonderful friends. Beth would be available to come down and work anytime. She was just a phone call and a ferry ride away. This was comforting for Debbie to know.

The support I received from patients was overwhelming. They were like my family. I was recently introduced to an extraordinary woman. Dr. Herman's partner, Dr. Cohen, referred her to my office when he learned of the MLD technique. Her name was Laura and she was truly an inspiration! She had a radical mastectomy over 20 years ago and she and her husband have shared a wonderful and fulfilling life together that includes two wonderful grandsons, and tons of traveling. Her life was a bit hampered with the edema she accumulated in her left arm from the mastectomy and I prayed to God that I could help her with that.

The pre-admissions tests went smoothly. It was a difficult day overall. My emotions stayed pretty well intact, but I could feel them banging on the door to come out. I knew the time was coming. When I returned home, the telephone was ringing. It was my OB/GYN doctor. I really had no desire to speak to him. I was still not over my reaction to him assuring me I was just cystic over the past year. Everybody was human and could make mistakes, but I had not completely forgiven him yet. I resented hearing his voice full of sympathy on the other end of the phone. I still cannot recall how the conversation ended. I became numb when he reassured me that he had many patients who were much worse off than I. Talk about being insensitive to your patient's feelings!

The phone had not been hung up for two seconds when it began to ring again. I exploded into tears. This was the beginning. My emotions would not be held back any longer. It was Robin, whom I adored. She was the nurse practitioner at our family doctor's office. She cried with me, and promised to come to the hospital to see me after the surgery. The phone rang again. This time it was Dr. Frazzano, our family doctor. He was very concerned and let me know that if I ever needed to talk, he would be there.

I felt so lucky to have all of these great people at my side. So, why couldn't I stop crying?

As soon as my composure was back intact, I phoned Dr. Barrall's office as I was told to do and spoke to his nurse, Cheryl. I broke down *again* and her response was immediate..."Linda, why don't you come right in and Dr. Barrall can talk to you and hopefully give you some peace of mind." I was grateful. I phoned Mike and assured him that I would be fine. I found Dr. Barrall's office with no difficulties.

Within minutes I was waiting in an exam room. Dr. Barrall entered through the door. I was surprised to see how young he was. I'm sure it was obvious that I'd been crying. Or he could have possibly thought that I had been out on a binge at a local bar. He began to speak first, describing the procedure for the type of reconstruction I would require. I tried so hard to speak, but instead those floods of tears began pouring again, uncontrollably. My temporary moratorium on emotions had just been lifted.

I was trying to tell him that I was not expecting to reproduce the breasts I had now. I could never do that. I was just looking for the smallest prosthesis to be inserted at the time of surgery. I don't think he heard a word I was saying. He probably couldn't believe that I was in the state of mind to be making these decisions. By now, I had totally saturated my sleeve with tears and runny nose. His examining room was not equipped for the sort of patient I was and neither was he. He very gracefully made his exit and sent in Cheryl with a box of tissue. She was so sweet.

Sitting next to me, she put her hand on my leg, "Linda, why don't you come back on Friday, in two days, and re-meet the doctor. It has been a very difficult day for you."

"Cheryl, he does not understand my needs. I just want two simple implants inserted at the time of surgery, not another surgery."

"I'll talk to him, and I'll also try to work out his patient schedule to accommodate your surgery." I agreed to return on Friday.

I got into my car, feeling as though I was the only lost soul on the planet. I plugged in my Stevie Winwood tape, since this was the surefire way to help me resolve the state of self pity I found myself falling into.

The incredible outburst of emotions I displayed shocked me. The timing was all wrong. The outburst was long overdue. I should have allowed myself my emotional reaction earlier when I felt it. Everything had been so rushed until now, with no time aside for just sitting and crying. I chose to have things move at a rapid pace. I knew I had already made most of my decisions. Now I was just following through with them, and it turned out to be happening very fast. I just wanted to keep my eyes open, looking for all of the open doors.

It was odd to me that people were treating me like I was ready to break apart under the slightest pressure. I don't think they believed that I was all right. I *was* being brave, and taking charge. I supposed they would catch on, sooner or later. If I had lived a life of wonderful dreams, I could better understand their behavior. But, most of these people have been aware of the contents of my life, and it hasn't always been pretty. I have taken the "course in bravery", and being born a Phelan certainly helps. The name itself means, "Brave As A Wolf." So my wonderful aunt swears that bravery is just an unavoidable, and blessed trait. I can't argue with that.

Deb canceled the appointments for the remainder of the day so that I could turn this terrible day into a brighter one. I wondered why I chose to go through this difficult day alone without emotional support. Maybe it was better this way. The closest I came to support was speaking to Mike on the phone. I asked if he would be disappointed if I chose not to seek out another plastic surgeon; that was, if Dr. Barrall was not able to perform the surgery.

Dead silence came over the phone. I despised that. He could say anything, but don't give me this silent act. I was certain that he was trying to come up with the most subtle way to express that he wanted the reconstruction. He finally spoke, almost in a saddened way, "Linda, I don't want you to do anything you don't want to do. If you think that having, or not having the reconstruction could make me love you any more, or any less, you're wrong. Seriously wrong."

I could feel his voice begin to tremble. We agreed that if it turned out that Dr. Barrall was not able to perform the surgery, for whatever reasons, I would not have it at all. All I knew was that I wanted this surgery done as soon as possible. The thought of any residual cancer cells swimming throughout my body made me crazy.

All my friends were very supportive, and the consensus was that the most important thing was certainly not having new boobs, but getting healthy again. I have to admit, though, I was praying that Dr. Barrall would agree to do the surgery...*my way* of course!

By the time Friday had come, I was worked into a frenzy. Meditation, visualization, herbal teas...nothing helped. I was so insecure about possible rejection from the initial impression Dr. Barrall may have gotten from me. After all, how many 29-year-old women has this surgeon consulted with regarding losing both breasts to cancer? I actually considered turning back and going home. But, I did the right thing, and reintroduced myself as the sane, intelligent woman that I am.

Dr. Barrall walked through the door as if it were the first time he was meeting me. Before I could say a word, he began speaking, "I have spoken to Dr. Herman, and he agreed that there should be enough skin left to successfully place two small silicone implants at the time of surgery. And my remarkable secretary/nurse has seen to it that I will be available to perform the surgery. So you must have impressed her because she doesn't do all that extra work for just anyone."

I thought I was going to cry for joy but managed to save it for later! He did ask me to agree to using expander bags if absolutely necessary. I did, but I knew he would do his best to place the implants then and there, even if it meant encouraging the nurses to have a tug-of-war with the leftover skin to make it stretch!

I never imagined that anybody could be so ecstatic under these circumstances. It showed me that circumstances did not decide the emotion—it came from within yourself, the most honest, simple truth of yourself. To find the good things out of the bad is surely an accomplishment. To be able to direct our vision through our hearts, eliminating the doubt and fear, gives us the power to override everything that is negative and find the positive—then we are in the right light.

CHAPTER 5

THE MAGIC OF THE STAR

In anticipation of the surgery, I was sending Dr. Barrall some pretty strong "thank you" vibes. Our next visit would be when I was on the table, under anesthesia. The thought of being put under...*ugh*! He would see me after the surgery and be the doctor in charge of my release. I thought it only fair to inform him that hospitals and I seem to have this love-hate relationship. He suggested that I focused on the love part since I should expect to be there for six days. Six days?! I laughed, and thought to myself, *sure*, six days. You better have some pretty heavy drugs to keep me there!

Being able to speak up on behalf of my needs, even under the most difficult of times, gave me a sense of empowerment. I really had been given some incredible strength for this. I played an important, participative role in the decision making process. The three of us, the two doctors and I, worked together. I felt very fortunate to have been guided to these two very special surgeons. They truly respected my role in my recovery.

It was such a terrific day, that I decided to check on the results from the liver and chest tests. I felt that they were both fine, and yes, I was right! Tomorrow would be the toughest day. Even though I felt certain that there were no other sites involved, I still remained intimidated by the bone scan.

I couldn't really figure it out. Maybe I was subconsciously reflecting back to my mother, since her cancer had metastasized there. I would have to work on resolving that issue to avoid any other interference.

On bone-scan day the forecast called for rain, and that only held one unfavorable memory for me. It had rained on the day of my biopsies. I decided this *must* be different. The girls were as excited about tagging the tree as I always was. So we piled in the car, and made our first stop at the hospital, arriving at the scheduled time of 9:00 a.m. It only took five minutes to inject the green goop into my veins. I felt like I could become invisible or something. Isn't that how the Teenage Mutant Ninja Turtles got so big? They were exposed to radioactive goop!

We drove out to the traditional Christmas Tree farm. I told the girls, "If we get separated, just look for the glow-in-the-dark figure!" We quickly chose a beautiful tree with lots of little pine cones still on it. With a real sense of satisfaction, we dropped the girls off at home and continued back to the hospital.

The gamma ray machine was every bit as intimidating as I had thought it would be. I lay under it for an hour while it scanned my entire body. Afterwards, I was asked to have a seat in the waiting area to be sure the films came out. When the technician appeared, with films in hand, I played the uneducated, silly woman hoping to sneak a peek at them. I don't know where that courage came from. She played to my stupidity and explained how the whole thing worked. She looked fairly pleased and I couldn't find any unusual sightings anywhere. The final sigh of relief would come after the radiologists report. Soon—I hoped.

My office was a welcomed haven for the few days before surgery. I gained a lot of strength from my supportive cast of friends and family. My Aunt Marge was very concerned. I think in her heart she knew all would be fine. But, being that distance away puts more emphasis on the worrying. I felt a great sense of love within me, and the power of prayer was present everywhere I turned. I prayed that I would know what route to take once the surgery was completed. I went to bed and looked out of my big bay window in the bedroom. There in the corner was a bright shining star. It was there to shine for me. The more I watched it, the brighter it sparkled.

"Life is a journey in the darkness if the night
Wake up to the inner light"

—The Mother
Pondicherry, India

How much do we really know about the universe? What about the dark matter. Why is it there with all those magnificent stars? Maybe when we leave our earth bodies, our spirits go into some sort of holding area. A star! We twinkle up there until our new lives are created. Free spirits, we're suspended in the outer most parts of space. I am not sure whose spirit my star carries. Whoever it is, they are very comforting.

I woke in the morning with a sense of decisiveness. I looked at Mike, who was standing over me and asked "So, do you think it will be the CMF or the CAF?" He just looked at me. Then I realized that I had just woken up with the decision made. I had chosen the next path and felt a sense of being very centered. Mike seemed happy and relieved.

Once the house was empty, with the girls at school, and Mike at work, I decided to take a nice bubble bath. Sort of a celebration. Not a usual thing for me to do in the morning. I normally take them at night to unwind and rethink the days events.

I lay in the tub and found myself very centered on my breath. A curious thing isn't it? Breath is something that happens quite naturally, like health. The rise and fall of every breath brings new life into us and lets the old out, how healing. It seems that my breath is translating the dialogue of my inner body. When I am upset, or tense, I can feel and see the rise and fall of my chest. I call this the stressed out breath. When I am calm, and relaxed, I can see and feel the breath in my abdomen, the center of our energy resides there.

Once my breath was relaxed, I began to focus it towards all the needed areas of my body, and actually, began the healing process without even being consciously aware of it. From that moment, I vowed to take on my full share of responsibilities for healing my body. The better portion, if not all of the healing process was in my hands. It makes perfect sense that if my body has produced this organic problem, why shouldn't it be able to get rid of it in the same way?

There is nothing synthetic about the human body. If disease is made within and from the by-products of the body's response to its environment, then why can't this process be reversed? The problem is all in our mind. If we can't see it, we don't believe it. Some of the most renown scientists and surgeons believe the body's own natural mechanisms can reverse disease.

This was how I decided to live. I would work with my body. So people asked, then why are you choosing to do chemotherapy? My only answer is that there is a best system for each person. I chose the best path to follow, for *me*. This I accepted. I was aware of the intensity of the event that was to take place soon, but it did not represent anything in my heart to fear. The removal of my breasts was not an issue. What real purpose did they serve? I had already nursed my children. Yes, they were a sensual tool, and could make sex a bit more interesting, but there was plenty where that came from. I found it difficult to think that this would change our already wonderful love life.

I am aware that many women experience insecurity, denial and even self hatred. I would never say anything to intentionally hurt someone else's feelings, but this is truly absurd. We are beautiful people, with or without breasts, legs, arms, or ovaries. What is real lives inside us. We can't see this with our eyes, but our eyes are only given to us for the material world. Our hearts and souls represent who we are, and we are all born beautiful. During those times when we may feel unloved, we must remember, we are forever loved by our Creator. It was out of His love that we exist. That love is unconditional, just like the love between a mother and child.

I took a long look in the mirror, and assured myself that I would continue to love and respect myself for as long as I was serving my purpose on this earth. After all, if we do not go into life with self love, where will it come from in the tough times? Love is a necessity for healing. As individuals, we have much to offer the world. I believe that if you live your life remaining in touch with the Infinite Power, you will experience yourself as a whole being. Body parts play no role in this.

When we are thrown off center, for whatever reasons (illness, financial, emotional, etc.), coming back to center brings us closer and closer to this wholeness. We must not see our mistakes as failures. Mistakes, just present us with another opportunity to achieve higher goals. To fail is to go down, and *stay* down for good. We would not expect the flower to bloom without giving it proper growing time along with lots of sun and water. Like the flower's cycle, every situation must come to a full circle before we can see results. There may be many pieces we need to complete our circle of growth, or there may be few. This depends on our individual path.

I saw my circle of health and harmony as consisting of 4 pieces. The first was cooperation between my mental, spiritual and physical selves. This included my: awareness, courage, optimism, meditation, prayer, inner searching, love, and faith. The second was my physical care: de-toxing, diet, supplements, exercise, spinal adjustments and work habits. The third was the actual surgery and elimination of the disease. The fourth was the adjunctive therapies like chemotherapy, to rid my body of any possible floating cells. These were all vital to my complete recovery. They would all have a curative effect if used in the proper ways.

My greatest source of comfort came from my horse. I sat in his stall for hours talking to him, and knowing he was listening. I took long bareback rides with him. He always knew how to respond to whatever was on my mind. Horses have as immense capacity to give love, and receive it. Their love is unconditional and so trusting. He snuggled his muzzle into my bosom and gave me every ounce of love that was within him, as I gave back to him.

> *"...the earth sings when he touches it;*
> *the basest horn of his hoofs is more musical than the pipes of Hermes...*
> *When bestride him I soar,*
> *I am a hawk..."*

—William Shakespeare

I began reading Shakti Gawain's *Creative Visualization* book. The more I read, the more of an illusion it seemed. I was not absorbing any of the information for some reason. The words seemed wonderful, so I thought, perhaps this just was not the right time for me to read it. I used my own images to visualize during stressful times, or times of healing.

I chose a strong, alert white wolf for my guide. I put him deep inside myself and there he stayed to help me along my journey. His keen eyes saw through my eyes. He gave me strength when I was weak, like a guardian. The white wolf represents everything that was masculine within myself.

I chose an iris to represent my feminine side. The iris within me grew more beautiful as it unfolded. It possessed the natural, healing shades of blue and purple, with white for purity. Its stem was long, thick and strong, rooted into the depths of my soul. I sought to grow like these wild irises, full of color and light.

Through each step of my recovery, I would bring into the process what I needed to learn and be guided by, to grow into my wholeness. This path was a long one and I asked only that I had the strength to climb the mountains, not that the mountains be moved from my path. This path shall be a formation of myself.

"The body should reject illness as energetically as in the mind we reject falsehood."

—The Mother
Pondicherry, India

The cards and calls of support were overwhelming. I had written my cousin in Germany with great apprehension. Gerd was very close to my mother and their relationship and bond were quite strong. I knew he would inform the rest of my family there, which would make things much simpler for me since I can't write in German.

The same day I entered this in my journal, I received a letter from Gerd. Our letters probably passed in the mail. He wrote to express his joy in the birth of a daughter! Gerd and his wife, Sabine, were in their forties and had tried for many years to have a child. They had finally given up hope, and now, shortly after the wall had been torn down, they were blessed with a daughter. He had not spoken a word to anyone about Sabine's pregnancy, due to the her possible difficulties. Although their daughter was born two months premature, she was fine. Her name was Christiane.

Reading Gerd's letter, I felt a terrible sinking feeling in my heart. I had sent a letter of unfortunate news at a time of joy in his life. I was so upset for interfering with his joy. That day I received a phone call from him. I spoke of joy for their new life, and he spoke of concern for mine. I assured him I would be fine and I knew he believed me. We would keep in touch.

Facing my surgery had been a cinch compared to what I had to do next. I needed to sit with Meg and somehow explain this difficult situation in five-year-old lingo. We sat on the couch and she looked up at me with that beautiful cherubic face of hers, "What's the matta, Mommy?"

"Well you see, honey, Mommy has some bad tissue in her breasts that has to come out. So I will have to be in the hospital for a few days where they can take extra special care of me. And you and Daddy and Cara can come visit me whenever you want to."

"Will it hurt you?"

"Oh no, not at all. You see they have this medicine that makes you fall asleep, and then they have another special medicine that wakes you up after, so you don't feel anything at all."

"OK Mommy. I'll take care of you." She was such a wonderful spirit. She smiled and said that I would be fine, and didn't display even the slightest bit of concern. I think children are deeply in touch with God. They are not complicated by the mind's twists and turns encountered in growing up. They convey a deep trust, and seem to have the most honest talks with God.

I pray a lot at night with Meg. She says the sweetest things, and I know those are things she would never say to just anyone. She really speaks to God. The only thing that remains the same in her prayers was the ending. I nearly cried the first time I heard her say it. She said, "And God, may you bless all of your wonderful living creatures, great and small. Amen." She covered about everything in that. I knew she was talking to God about me, and he was giving her reassurance. I kissed her little cherubic face one-hundred times.

Cara was eight years older. I remember watching my mother die when I was her age. She was aware of my experience. Cara needed her space and I respected her. When she needed me to be with her, she knew I would be there. I knew she had a lot of people who offered to talk, and counsel was available for her. She would think about it. She was aware of her resources, and that knowledge alone comforted her.

Mike was expecting her to come to him in her times of need. I was sure that this wouldn't happen. I could have never spoken to my father about my concerns. It would have been impossible for him to understand where my emotions were coming from, and unfair of me to expect him to. Cara and Mike would experience different feelings, but of course would always be there for one another.

My friends and family no longer concealed their worrisome faces. I seemed to be the only one, aside from Meghan, who was calm and relaxed. I found myself falling into the role of their supporter. There has been so much prayer said for me over the past weeks that I can feel the added strength when I pray. During a time like this, everyone asks if there was anything they could do. This offer should never be turned down. No matter what religion, people can pray for you. I have found more peace in this than I could even begin to express.

My dear friend Steve, a chiropractor, encouraged me to see him for an alignment before the surgery. We spoke briefly. He said, "The one thing besides my friendship and caring that I can give you is my talent. I would really like for you to be treated frequently during your chemotherapy. There are several nerves that exit the spinal column between every vertebrae and these nerves are responsible for getting blood and oxygen to their designated areas in your body. If your spine is out of alignment the nerves and blood vessels become pinched off, the areas supplied by these vessels are starved of their much needed nourishment." Steve felt this was especially true during chemotherapy when my muscles would be weak, and unable to give strong support to the skeletal system.

This was his gift to me and I accepted it thankfully. Steve also provided an endless supply of magnificent hugs, both before and after each adjustment. What a deal! I always said that if he ever became unable to perform his duties as a chiropractor, he could probably do the world every bit as good, sitting on a street corner and giving hugs. He's a great hugger.

Andrea brought over two flannel button-down night shirts she had bought. She knew that there was a very slim chance that I would be caught with a hospital gown on. This was hard for her. She had watched her mother succumb to breast cancer yet she still chose to involve herself with my life and disease. She was quite motherly and had a lot of spiritual strength.

Kevin expressed a desire to visit me in the hospital. What a surprise! He likes hospitals about as much as I do—not much. I couldn't resist his offer and I was sure he knew how good it would make me feel. I asked if he could bring one of his cassette Walkmans when he came so that I could easily escape into my music. He was honored to do so. Jeff had already decided that he would like to come with us to the hospital and keep Mike company. I suppose misery loves company. I agreed that it was a good idea. It would make Jeff feel useful.

For the second time, I tried to get the results on the bone scan with no success. This began to frighten me. Was this because they didn't want to stress me any more than necessary before the surgery? My head felt like a water balloon ready to explode if I had one more thought about the bone scan. It was out of my hands. I would just have to be patient, not one of my best virtues.

I felt the pressure of surgery drawing near. Mike and I stayed up quite late sharing our feelings. I wasn't making any jokes now. It's true, I did fear the anesthesia more than anything tomorrow. I said, "I want to talk about what I'd like for you to do just in case I don't wake up. After all, some people are so content to be put wherever that anesthesia puts you that they decide not to come back."

"Don't expect me to laugh about this Linda," he said, "but you're right, we should talk."

"I can't stand the thought of being buried. It really terrifies me, so make sure I get cremated, OK? No wake or funeral unless it is just for our immediate family and friends, but definitely no make-up. I would like an intimate gathering of friends and family. They have to wear at least one piece of clothing that is purple. Be sure to play my favorite music since I will be somewhere in the room dancing with you all one last time.

"Now, with my life insurance, I would like you to hire a woman to be around to clean, iron and be here when the girls come home. And she *must* be at least fifty years old and fifty pounds overweight. You don't need any distractions. Always talk about me so the girls remember me, and try not to remarry for at least a year...preferably five!"

He couldn't contain himself any longer. "What if this fifty-year-old comes from Sweden, what is she going to do with her twenty-five-year-old daughter? She can't just leave her in Sweden. Can she come too?" We laughed and we cried. We made some of our most memorable love that night. We held each other tightly and wished each other a good night. I stayed, lying there in his arms, watching my star in the corner of the window, smiling at me. I began to cry a soft quiet cry.

I somehow knew that my guardian angel was sitting upon that star watching me. I envisioned her guiding me along my difficult path to a place of greatness and joy—where I need not go looking for happiness, and peace and love would surround me like the air I breathe.

CHAPTER 6

JOURNEYING THROUGH THE OUTER

I must have needed to cry those last few tears in private, but come morning I was full of energy, strength and courage.

Jeff arrived and he helped us get the girls off to school. I kissed and hugged Meg. She held me in her tiny embrace for a moment and looked at me, "Mommy, the doctors will take good care of you and I promise the pinch-pinch won't hurt." This was something I told her in the past while on Tegretol. She had to have her blood work done every six weeks and she was always a brave little Indian about it.

I took Cara's hand since it was obvious that she was not comfortable with exchanging hugs. She was scared to death. I could see it in her eyes. "Cara, always remember how wonderful life is, even in the midst of a crisis. If you keep sight of this, you will keep your enthusiasm for life."

Cara squeezed my hand and without making eye contact said, "I love you, Mom." Plans for my surgery had been shared with the school. The staff was very supportive and prepared to assist the girls in any way they could.

I packed up my small bags with a few necessities and made sure I didn't forget my lucky socks. They would have to knock me out to get them off of me! I felt somewhat invisible to the two important men in my life. They exchanged some conversation between themselves but said nothing to me. I decided to allow them this freedom, to deal with the situation in any way that would make them comfortable. I sat and prayed silently. We were directed to a waiting area. Jeff asked, "Are you nervous?"

"A bit, but nothing compared to what I had expected." A very pleasant nurse called my name and showed me to a dressing room where I changed into my chic gown. I sat in a recliner and waited briefly until Michael and Jeff walked in. I had this great sense of calm about me. I only wished I could say the same for them. I didn't have the heart to insult their integrity by saying, "What's the matter with you fools?" I was the one who was supposed to be nervous. But, they would be the ones pacing the floor while I was out cold.

The nurse excused them while she prepped me for the trip down the hall. I graciously received two shots, one in each cheek. I don't know why but these seem to be the most painful and humiliating. They were ready to take me, so Mike was called into the room to give me a smooch.

I wanted to cry for Mike. I felt like I was looking into the young face of a boy. He was holding the tears back with all his might. I thought, this was what my own father must have felt, this awful sense of helplessness. What could I do? I couldn't imagine him sitting out there with Jeff just waiting. Then, a wonderful thought dropped into my brain, "Mike, would you like to know what I would really love for you to do?" He looked relieved. I was about to give him orders. The only time in his life that his ears perked like a dog's to get orders.

"I would be so happy if you would go to the barn and lunge the horse since he hasn't had any exercise in a week!" He happily agreed. Meanwhile the nurses were all waiting for an explanation of exactly what I had just asked my husband to do. I explained to them that it meant putting the horse on a long rope and letting him run around in circles, because Mike does not ride. They all laughed and Mike felt a whole hell of a lot better. The nurse assured him that Dr. Herman would call as soon as his job was completed and Dr. Barrall took over.

Mike leaned over the stretcher and said, "Do you know how much I love you?"

"I think so, but please keep reminding me, OK?" He kissed me and smiled. Thank you, God. I knew the horse would give him the support and deep understanding that all animals give, and that Ritchie, the barn owner, would be there to lend support. Mike needed the right energy sources to draw from. *Banded*, my horse, knew that there was something unusual going on since I had spent several hours with him the week before, crying and laughing. He would enjoy Mike's company. "Please tell Jeff I love him, and I will be fine," I added, as he was walking through the doors to leave. Dr. Herman's surgery was scheduled to take no more than three hours and he would phone Mike then. The entire surgery was to take about five hours.

So, as we shoved these two grown men out the door to go play with the horse, I was wheeled down the hall. We took the scenic route through the putrid blue corridors, and a free trip on the elevator. I was told that I was in the holding area. I thought, "No way...this isn't the dark blue sky, and I certainly don't look like a star." The drugs were kicking in. I looked around in hopes of seeing Dr. Herman. I wanted to give him an unforgettable hug and tell him it was in anticipation of a job well done. Nothing like putting a little pressure on the man. I kept looking and repeating what I wanted to say in my head.

The next thing I knew, I was lying on a bed, with the breathing tube still in my throat. This panicked me. I thought, oh my God, am I waking up during the surgery? Normally, this was not something you remembered, since they got that damn tube out of your throat before you were totally conscious. I thought I was being a bit stubborn about breathing on my own as I was coming out of anesthesia. My eyes were filled with water.

I had an excruciating pain in the middle of my back on the right side. It felt like they had operated there since I really didn't have any sensation in my chest. The nurse kept prodding me to open my eyes. I wanted to say, "Stop pouring water over my face and I will gladly open them!" I could only manage opening one eye at a time. It seemed impossible to open both of them.

I heard the nurse call Mike's name. He was walking in and the nurse began joking about the one eye bit. I wanted to ask him to plow her one, but instead asked for a kiss. He was shaking. I remember nothing after that, but learned later that the nurse asked me if I had ever had Demoral before and I replied, "Oh yes!" She then asked me if I would like a shot and I dittoed that reply. What a time to ask someone a question like that! Of course I was going to take the shot! I woke at 10:00 p.m., all tucked into my bed in my room.

Within five minutes of opening my eyes, a nurse came quietly tip-toeing in with another needle. She said I am here to give you another shot of Demerol. "Are you all right?"

I said, " Yes, but this pain in my back is excruciating," which was why I agreed to have the shot.

She leaned over to roll me onto my side a bit and said, "I'm sorry if this hurts you, but I just have to move you a little so that I can reach your buttocks!" My chest was a bit sore, but nothing that required pain medication. Afterwards, she tucked me back in and said, "I'll be back in to give you a back rub since you're awake." I thought, oh yes, that would be great. I realized that it was probably ordered by the surgeon, in order to stimulate the flow of everything.

The nurse came in with a small bottle of cream and said, "Now I need to position you again." I made every effort to accommodate her in anticipation of a soothing, nurturing back massage. She proceeded to rub the lotion on my back. What I thought was a brief stop to put more cream on was actually the end of the massage.

I was amazed. "You know, when I get well, I will come back here and teach you how to give a real massage!" She chuckled, unaware that this was my area of expertise. I dozed back to slumberland. I woke at 2:00 a.m. to find another nurse sneaking into my room with a flashlight. When she noticed that I was awake, she said she used the flashlight so that she wouldn't wake me. Good thing, I was beginning to wonder. She had another shot. Before she could speak I said, "I would prefer to not have the shot, but I would appreciate some oral medication".

She said, "I'm sorry but I cannot dispense any oral medication without the doctors orders." I asked her what time Dr. Barrall and Herman would be coming. She said Dr. Herman usually makes his rounds early. She was not sure about Dr. Barrall. I said I would wait for Dr. Herman and assured her that if I was in pain, and reconsidered, she would be the first to know.

She left the room and it was then that I noticed the two small, but very distinct, bumps all bandaged up. Thank You!! I got my bumps! What a feeling. And they even looked pretty. I noticed that I was hooked up to two large suction containers on the wall which was taking the blood and lymph fluid out from under the implants. I had four tubes coming out from the bandages—two on each side. I still had the catheter in place. That would be the *first* thing to go in the morning. I was grateful that I didn't remember a thing about the operating room, but still upset about not giving Dr. Herman his hug. I'm sure he did a terrific job anyway.

The pain in my back was really beginning to get to me. I decided it must have been from having my arms strapped up during the surgery. That would do it. I could feel the spasms in my back. I was happy that Beth was due out from the Vineyard today. She was going to a Bernie Siegel lecture in Boston that we had planned to go to together, long before any of this came up. She was going to tape it for me. She also wanted to massage my arms and legs. I meditated for a while and thought about seeing my beautiful girls and wonderful husband later on.

At 6:30 a.m., Dr. Herman presented himself in my room. I was never so happy to see him. His face was alive, and I was happy to see his bright face and balding head that shone like his eyes. "You look terrific," he said.

"Oh, I'll bet you say that to everyone," I replied.

"I wrote you an order for pain medication so you can have it whenever you would like."

"Lets talk about the outcome of the surgery first," I said.

He sat on my bed, still smiling, "It all went fine."

"I never got to see you before the surgery, and I wanted so bad to give you a hug in anticipation of a job well done!"

"Linda, you're the first patient that has ever hugged me *before* the surgery."

"What? I don't remember seeing you."

"That's because of the medication they gave you. It has an amnesiac effect."

"My God, what else did I do or say in there." The grin on his face said it all. I blushed.

"Oh no, don't worry, you didn't give away any secrets or anything!" He said the surgery went fine but it took longer than expected. I did quite a lot of bleeding, mostly due to my age and the heavy blood supply to the chest wall. Dr. Barrall had his hands full trying to insert the prosthesis through all of the bleeding. He didn't feel the need for me to receive a transfusion, thank goodness. My blood counts were low but he had every faith that I would eat properly and take my iron to bring them back up. I would experience some fatigue until this was accomplished.

Dr. Herman explained what the scar would look like. He had to make a vertical incision for about two inches, to clean out the area of the large tumor on the right breast that would leave an additional scar. I was not at all shook up over that bit of news. He removed the nodes, and the results would probably be out in a week. I asked about the bone scan, remembering I still had access to that Demoral needle if I needed it. He promised to find out the results today. With that he left, promising to see me later.

The morning nurse brought in the pain medication. Her name was also Linda and she was very young and very pretty. Her family was from Bristol and owned the grinder shop that we frequently went to. I begged and pleaded with her to remove the catheter. "Well, why not?" she said. So I went into position, and out it came. I still had an IV needle in my hand which was pumping fluid and antibiotics into me. "I can't remove that one Linda, sorry. You have to be drinking enough water on your own before they will allow me to remove it." I couldn't argue with her. She was so sincere and sympathetic that I could only be grateful to have her for my nurse.

Mike came in at eight-thirty. It was so great to see him. He looked a little rough around the edges. Overall he seemed to have handled everything all right and successfully got the girls off to school. We joked around about the look of confusion that came over the nurse's faces when I asked Mike to lunge the horse. It was nice to laugh with him.

Mike said he spent about two and a half hours with Banded and Ritchie and that I was right, it really helped to soothe him. Jeff reluctantly went home. After the quality horse time, Mike decided he'd better get home and wait for Dr. Herman's call. Then three hours passed. At three and a half hours, the girls came home. He was about to call the hospital, when the phone rang. It was Dr. Herman saying that he had finished up and Dr. Barrall was taking over.

Dr. Barrall would also phone Mike upon his completion so that by the time he got up there, he would be able to see me. He waited and waited. After seven hours, he was really beginning to sweat. Finally, the phone rang and Dr. Barrall said that everything was fine, and explained that the bleeding slowed things down quite a bit—two extra hours in surgery! I nearly fainted. We joked about the one eye bit and the Demoral. I told him how worried I was for him when he left the hospital, and how I spoke to God and asked him to help you while I was being rolled down the lovely blue corridors.

> *"He giveth power to the faint: and to them that have no might, he increaseth strength."*

—Isaiah 40:29

Mike could see the pain in my face and thought it was my chest hurting. I told him about the pain in my back and we both agreed on the cause. He sat me up just enough so that he could get his hand back there and as soon as he touched it, I thought I was going to vomit. It was like someone jabbing a fine blade into my back. I had to ask him to stop. Mike hadn't heard anything about the bone scan, but was every bit as curious as I was. I said the lymph nodes would take about a week and he seemed comfortable with that.

Dr. Barrall strolled in, lively and chipper, around 9:30 a.m. "Oh thank you for giving me my implants," I beamed!

"I'm just happy that we could do it for you. I realized just how much it meant to you." He stood above the bed, taller than any of my other doctors, about six feet three inches. I noticed that for a man of his size, he was very light on his feet. Dr. Herman takes heavy steps, like a man on a mission.

"So my surgery took double time? I hope it didn't interfere with any plans of yours? I was having visions of nurses tugging on my left over skin." He just laughed, "I had to irrigate you a lot during the procedure. Every time I picked up the muscle flap to insert the implant, you would bleed."

"I wouldn't be surprised if one bump was down around my belly button and the other up near my chin." He laughed. They came out pretty well he thought. Of course I will have some discomfort in my back for a while since the tissue and muscles are being pulled, and having to make some major adjustments to accommodate the prosthesis. I assured him that he was correct about the pain in the back, but that Beth would be there soon to work on that, if he didn't mind. He approved, but recommended I be kept quiet. I did my best to dazzle him with a smile and asked about the IV needle.

He asked, "Are you drinking enough?"

"Oh yes, tons!"

"Maybe tomorrow, I'll have to leave the needle in, though, so we can hook you up to antibiotics every four hours." That sounded reasonable to me, at least for now. "The suction is mandatory, but when the amount of fluid is reduced to an acceptable level, we'll disconnect the automatic suction and put you on self-suction. These are little balls that resemble hand grenades at the end of each tube. These just need to be squeezed before they are closed and that will maintain an acceptable amount of suction." I was sure that I would progress rapidly along this plan.

Mike helped me wash up and put on one of my new night shirts. I even slipped on my white cotton bike shorts for a little added comfort. I felt like a new person after I brushed my teeth and put on a pair of amethyst earrings. Amethysts are good healing stones. Mike had bought several things for me from my favorite shop in Newport called *Portobello*. They have the best jewelry, with a lot of reproduction work.

To my surprise, my lucky socks had managed to stay on my feet. Linda had to take them off to put on a pair of those ever so fashionable anti-blood-clotting stockings. Not even in my color. But, the worst thing was they were made of some synthetic garbage. If it wasn't cotton, it didn't touch my feet. Oh well, this would have to be one of the few exceptions.

Beth arrived shortly after my wardrobe change. My heart was grateful for her soft, subtle presence. She seemed to smile at me with her entire body. "I am so happy to see you, Linda! And I love your outfit. You realize you are a perfect example of Bernie Siegel's *Bad Patient*, not capitulating to all the hospital rules. But, of course, those are the signs of a survivor! Can I hug you or will I hurt you?"

"Oh, please hug me!" I have such tremendous respect and love for her.

"I can tell you're in pain. What can I do to help you"?

"I think you could touch any part of my body and it would sigh with relief, but I suppose we should pay some attention to this little knife that has been piercing my back since I woke up last night."

"Sure," Beth smiled. With that, she took a deep breath and focused her entire mind on my back, zeroing right in on the problem. I realized that our friendship was just beginning. We would become more bonded with each passing year. We first met in massage school and had the perfect opportunity to develop our friendship through touch and conversation. I could imagine having some sort of connection with her in a previous lifetime, perhaps. Friendship was one of those gifts from God that you didn't remember asking for. It was a gift that required no reciprocation, only understanding.

There were no signs of swelling in my arms and I was very happy about that. I realized, however, from the patients that I treated, that swelling could come about quite unexpectedly with no known cause. But, surgery was a major cause of edema.

The flowers were beginning to take up the whole room. They were all so beautiful. Mike brought irises! I was only a little disappointed when he couldn't find a white wolf! Flowers came from my patients, friends, family, and even people Mike works with who I have never met. As I lay there, in the silent companionship that filled the room, the beauty of the irises filled my mind with peace.

It was time for Beth to leave so that she could beat the traffic into Boston. "I promise that I will be back on the return trip, sometime Sunday. That is, of course, if you haven't fought your way out of here by then!" Mike left to run some errands before going home to greet the girls, and I looked forward to some quiet time to read.

As I opened my book, my brother Kevin and his wife Mary walked through the door. They are a beautiful couple. Kevin was larger than life and incredibly like my father, while Mary was so light and unpretentious. They were horrified by the suction and all the IV paraphernalia, but I assured them, "It looks much worse than it really is."

"Hey there, how ya doin?" Kevin's words struck me. Obviously he was reaching for something to say. A ludicrous situation for a Phelan!

"Never mind me, how are the two of you doing in the setting you dread most?"

"Fine," they replied almost simultaneously.

"This is a great hospital!" Kevin sounded enthusiastic, "Small enough so that it does not seem so intimidating. We brought you the Walkman you wanted, and we even picked out some tapes for you. I knew you loved Steve Winwood and we grabbed a few more," he said. Mary began unwrapping the Walkman and tapes.

"Kevin, I just asked to borrow one of yours. You didn't have to run out and spend money."

"Hey, what are brothers for?" he said. It's so typical for Phelans to overdo a situation. Generosity was our middle name and I must admit I wouldn't have wanted it any other way.

"Thank you Kev, that was very sweet of you." I must have shown some signs of fatigue since in no time they were standing up to say their good-byes so that I could get some rest.

Mary slowly walked over to my bed, "I thought you might like to read this book by Joseph Campbell, *The Power Of Myth*." I thanked her as she bent over my bed and kissed my forehead. It reminded me of the soft kiss of a mother, tenderly kissing her sick child's forehead. Sort of a non-verbal way of saying "heal". I wanted to cry. Kevin then kissed me and gave me that concerned, brotherly look.

I tried to comfort them, "I will be out of here soon, very soon." They left and I cried. I missed them being a part of my life but could feel that the situation would change soon. This cancer experience was creating an entirely new and stronger bond between us all. I have never had such a strong sense of family. I feel that so much depends on them right now. Not in an individual sense, but in a whole sense.

As badly as I wanted to rest, I was glad to see Dr. Herman come in. He was smiling even more than usual, "Your bone scan is fine! I apologize for the delay in the reading. I'm not sure what happened, but I wanted to give you that news right away."

I gave him a grateful hug which nearly sent my suction into a frenzy, "Now how about the lymph node report? Is there any way to speed that up?"

"I wish I could Linda, but some things we just have to be patient about."

"If I hold you for ransom, do you think it might give them some incentive to hurry it up?" He gave me a hug of reassurance and left the room with the same determination I always feel in his movement. I'm glad he's my doctor.

My doctors seemed to be in sync with one another, for as soon as he disappeared, Dr. Barrall appeared. Not quite as comfortable with patient intimacy, he stood a short distance away from me, but was always very polite and sincere.

"How are you feeling?"

"I feel like I could dismiss all of this hospital paraphernalia, and feel much better." He smiled. I said, "I am willing to beg if need be, but I would rather not have to resort to that sort of adolescent behavior."

"Let me see how much fluid is coming out with the suction." He leaned over and I could see in his face that he was satisfied. "OK Linda, you win. I will have your nurse come in and detach the suction. I'll be by to see you in the morning, and by the way, you look great in your outfit."

"So good that I don't need the IV anymore?" I pressed. He laughed.

"Maybe tomorrow we can see about that, but humor me until then, OK?" Fair enough, I thought to myself. Tomorrow it will be. I was truly living up to the "Bad Patient" standards. He fidgeted around sort of randomly before gliding out the door. Again, I listened but could not here his footsteps. I put on my Steve Winwood tape, lay back and smiled. There has never been a time when a Steve Winwood song didn't make me smile. *Back In The High Life* seemed an appropriate song, since I knew it would apply to me in the next year. It's wonderful the way music can give you such a feeling of comfort and joy simply through a combination of words and sounds.

Rosemary hadn't phoned me yet, so I thought I'd call her and let her know that all was well. I also needed to phone Karen, my angel, who knew all along I'd be taken care of. When the wonderful gourmet hospital food arrived, I traded it for my raisins and juice.

I got up to brush my teeth and noticed my forehead had a dark red mark across it. Just then, Mike phoned to say that he wouldn't be coming up. I asked him about the red mark and he said it was there since I was in recovery. I thought that my guardian angel must have been rubbing my forehead reassuringly, like the kiss I had received earlier from Mary. Since my guardian angel had to rub for over seven hours, the mark was unavoidable. Mike was just silent. He must have thought I had accepted another shot of Demoral.

"Cara is not up to coming to the hospital," he said quietly. I felt my heart sink immediately, then remembered how difficult it was to see my own mother confined to a hospital bed. I could feel exactly what it was she was feeling.

"I understand, honey. It is very hard for her to see me like this. Meg, on the other hand, will think it nothing less than fascinating to see all the tubes, blood and wires! Why don't we just leave the girls alone and I will see them when I come home. This floor is a bit depressing, anyway, and I would hate for them to have a negative memory of this."

"OK, then I will see you in the morning?"

"I'll be here. By the way, Dr. Barrall says that I will be needing a size 34 cotton bra before I leave the hospital. Would you mind a little shopping before you come up?"

"Not at all," Mike laughed, "My pleasure." I could just imagine the fun he would have searching through all sizes and shapes.

I hung up the phone and began reflecting on the recent death across the hall. An older woman was brought in who was terrified of death and dying. I could hear it in her cries. I never heard any of the several people who entered her room speak. It was as if every moment of her life added to her crying and pain. I felt that she deserved a peaceful death after living such a long life. All of the emotional tugging to keep her alive was denying her a peaceful passage. I wanted to hold her hand and give her the reassurance she needed to let go, but I was too drugged and attached to tubes. Finally, her family left and a nurse went in to be with her. Within ten minutes, she stopped crying and died peacefully.

I wondered why death had to be so difficult. Birth was so joyous, and death so sad. Shouldn't we be allowed to leave with the same love and comfort that we entered with? When we could embrace death as simply another aspect of the life cycle, we would be able to appreciate and value each life encounter fully, knowing that it would never occur in the same way again. Perhaps the fact of life most conducive to living fully as a person was an honest awareness and acceptance of death.

That night passed well. I did read and listened to some music. Around six in the morning, I woke, half expecting Dr. Herman's smile to beam in at any minute. I made sure my hair was combed and my earrings were in. His beam of light preceded him through the door! "Linda, you look radiant." I could feel my face flushing! "This is the face I will see on a book."

"Did you know I was keeping a journal?" I asked.

"No, but that's terrific. What I do remember is how disgusted you were when you were searching the bookstores looking for something written by a younger breast cancer survivor and couldn't find anything." Ah yes, I remembered.

"So really, how are you feeling?"

"Terrific! I can't explain it, but I feel vibrant and healthy, and completely healed. I have managed to convince Dr. Barrall to disconnect me from all this machinery."

"I'm not surprised Linda. I think if you put your mind to it, you could do just about anything. I'll be by in the morning to see your lovely face!" Breakfast was wheeled in and without thinking, I popped my vitamins into my mouth. I was not sneaky enough to go unnoticed by Dr. Herman. I explained firmly that these were just some supplements and no matter what anyone said, I was going to take them. He closed his eyes and with his ever so determined way, left the room.

I have always been interested in vitamins. Since my diagnosis, I had read a great deal about vitamin therapy and cancer. Cancer was often caused by a basic mechanism of growth in the body which had lost the ability to be controlled. I found that vitamins could provide building blocks that were essential to repairing many of those mechanisms. Based on my reading, I took a specific dosage of vitamins A, C, E, and selenium, along with enzymes to help utilize proteins. I planned to take them faithfully for the rest of my life.

I also planned to drink fresh carrot juice every day. Carrot juice has a high concentration of electrified vitamin A, meaning it's in a form already available for the body's use. So much information was coming out on cancer and nutrition, I thought anybody with this disease should be carefully thinking about what they ate.

My nurse came in with a rather concerned look on her face. "Are you all right?" I asked.

"I'm fine, Linda, but Donna, another patient of Dr. Barrall's down the hall, is scheduled for surgery in a few hours and is emotionally devastated. Do you think there is any way you could talk to her?" Before she completed the sentence, I was working my way off the bed. She disconnected me from the suction and gave me a crash course on how to close the self-sucking grenades. Then she removed the IV attachment, and I was rolling. I put on some slippers and trotted down the hall to Donna's room. There she was, looking as terrified and vulnerable as I must have. I introduced myself and told her a little about my successful surgery. I knew she would be pleased with Dr. Barrall but I was unfamiliar with her surgeon.

"Regardless," I comforted her, "everything will be fine. I will say a prayer for you." Her face lit up with gratitude and she seemed to find some peace. I held her hand, "I promise to be watching for you later on, and visit again when you are up to it."

I went back and prayed for her, requesting the same lovely angel that reassuringly patted my forehead do the same for her. Back in my room I collapsed onto my bed like I just completed a ten mile road race! Exhilarated, I lay there with my eyes closed and peaceful.

By the time I opened my eyes, Dr. Barrall was there, "Thank you for speaking to Donna, Linda. I think it helped her." He checked the suction and the IV needle.

Then I got really gutsy, "Why can't I take oral antibiotics? I thought he was going to suspend me from the hospital and regret ever meeting me. I was wrong. Fortunately, he understood my need to have a little control.

"I think that I could arrange that." Hurray! Was it finally time to hug him? No, I thought. I didn't want to get him all shook up before his surgery with Donna. "Where is your husband this morning?" he asked.

"Well he is on a quest for the perfect 100% cotton post-mastectomy bra."

"Gee," he smiled, "I can't wait to see what he comes back with." Within minutes after he left, my nurse came in and removed the IV. *Good riddance!*

The oncologist, Dr. Strair, came in for an unexpected visit, "I think you made the right decision in having the mastectomies, Linda. As it turns out, you had other sites of cancer. It looks like five in all. Three in the right breast and two in the left." I was speechless. They were small sites, but just the same they were cancerous.

Jeff called to say he and Linda would be up to visit this evening along with my Aunt Kay. Aunt Kay was very worried about me. Mike was nowhere to be found and it was nearing 12:00 noon. Finally a collect call came in from him. He was out shopping in lingerie departments. This couldn't be. They must have the wrong number.

"Truly," he said, "all these woman think that I am just being naive when I ask for an all-cotton bra. They insist on dangling lacy satin sexpot material in front of my face, thinking this is really what I am looking for." I never thought I would hear him complain of such a thing. He said he had been everywhere except for CWT's in the mall.

Trying to keep my voice serious I told him, "Go into the CWT lingerie department, and tell the woman straight out that your wife is in the hospital, following mastectomy surgery for cancer. It's her surgeon's recommendation that she only wear an all-cotton bra. Could you please show me what is available in a 34A."

"OK, I think I can remember that. I'll be there as soon as I can."

I hung up the phone and told Linda, my nurse, and we both rolled with laughter. She smiled, "Well, if he is out buying you lingerie and you are expecting guests, I better get the dry shampoo and do your hair." What a peach. In most places, you would have to beg and plead for a nice shampoo, but not here, and not with Linda. With clean hair, I felt like a new person. I changed into my blue night shirt and fresh cotton socks.

Mike finally arrived looking like he had been dragged through the lingerie mill. He made a fine selection though. He even bought me a new *norfin*, better known as a troll. I loved them as a little girl, and every Christmas the girls buy me a new one. I have a hillbilly girl and boy, and a bride and groom. Mike bought me a surgeon, all dressed up in scrubs, so cute! I asked him which surgeon it was supposed to resemble. He said he hadn't thought of it, but which ever I decided would be fine. He brought some delicious lentil soup that Beth had brought down with her. The soup should help with my blood problem because lentils are high in iron.

Mike helped me distribute some flowers around the floor. We took some across the hall where a young woman was resting with a ton of equipment surrounding her. She had half of her lung removed from cancer. She couldn't speak, but she smiled at me. I set a basket up on Donna's table for her to see when she opened her eyes. I met her private duty nurse who her husband had hired. I wanted to tell him it wasn't necessary, to save his money because the nurses here were wonderful, but knew it wasn't my business. Mike had to leave to get the girls off the bus, so he kissed me and agreed to phone this evening. Tomorrow was Saturday so he wasn't sure what time he would be up to visit. I began to read some more of *The Power Of Myth*. Fascinating book.

Our family nurse practitioner, Robin, arrived. I had forgotten about her wanting to visit. "You don't know how happy I am to see how well you are doing," she greeted me.

"What's really terrific is that my insides feel as jubilant as the outside!" We hugged each other. I told her the story about Mike and laughed just as hard telling it the second time. Robin noticed my journal on the bed and inquired. Karen had given me a beautiful journal for writing, remembering how therapeutic it had been for her. I said that it was a healthy way of digesting things in my mind and working out worries. By expressing my anger on paper, I could read it and reread it until I was ready to put it behind me. Robin agreed. She asked me to call her and set up a lunch date with her once I felt up to it. I promised I would do just that.

Donna was out of surgery, but I knew that she wouldn't be up to any visitors until tomorrow. I did see her husband, with the same worried look on his face that I had seen on Mike.

I was soon busy with a round of visitors. Andrea and her wonderful husband, Joe, came for a short visit. I was happy to see them and told them how grateful I felt to be blessed with so many wonderful friends. Jeff, Linda and my Aunt Kay arrived next. Andrea and Joe greeted them and left, since my room could barely accommodate four guests at a time. I was tickled to see their surprise at finding me sitting there, all groomed and looking fine, especially Jeff. My Aunt was truly dumbfounded.

Before long, Dr. Barrall made his final rounds for the evening. My Aunt was astonished at how young he was. He looked modestly embarrassed, but got right to business, "Linda, we have decided that all this improvement deserves a reward. How would you like to go home tomorrow?" I was too shocked to remember to make a smart remark.

I was so thrilled at the thought of being home with my family, that I jumped right off the bed with excitement. I was anxious to see Meg's bony knees and Cara's warm eyes. I longed to place my hands over her soft round breasts and bless them, to somehow keep them safe. Dr. Barrall said he would return in 15 minutes to remove my bandages. My company was suddenly eager to leave. I invited all of them to stay for the unveiling, but I had no takers. Instead, Jeff agreed to see me at home.

Dr. Barrall entered the room with all the necessary instruments for the memorable moment. He stood back and asked calmly, "Are you ready?"

"What? Of course I'm ready. Would you prefer me to do the honors?"

He chuckled, "That's my privilege." We talked about the apprehensions many woman have at this moment, and how many even refuse to look at themselves.

"Not this one."

"I should have realized that without asking." Right. "Expect it to be swollen for a while Linda. I would like to remove the drains next Wednesday, this way they will have been in for a full week." Clip, clip, clip, the cutting began. I still marvel at what medicine can do. I had two perfect bumps. While he was cutting, I told him the story of the bra. He thought the bra was perfect. "I think Mike should be elected as the designated bra purchaser for all my patients."

"I don't think he could stand the stress of it. But, thanks for the offer!"

Dr. Barrall helped me with the bra. I still had one strip of bandage across the scar. He explained that this will probably stay on until I saw him on Friday, when they would remove the external sutures. He explained most of the sutures were internal, except across the sternum, where it was very tight and he had to use external sutures. I thought it was time to present him with his much deserved hug. It went well, better than I expected. I thanked him from the bottom of my heart, and he looked obviously flattered by my words. He promised to be in again in the morning to release me. They were such sweet words to hear after only two days!

I phoned Mike and he couldn't believe what I was saying. Yes, yes, of course he would be there first thing, 9:00 a.m. sharp to pick up his wife and her floral collection. I asked Mike to bring an outfit that wouldn't compress the drains to much...something loose fitting. I knew Cara would be the one to pick something out. Phoning everyone I knew, I spread the great news. Everyone was thrilled that I succeeded in getting evicted. I thanked God, and my wonderful nurse, Linda. I don't know how I managed to fall asleep, but I did.

By morning, I was washed up and shining. I was stunned to see both doctors in my room at the same time, a special occasion. Dr. Herman noticed my troll on the night stand, "So which one of us is it supposed to be, Linda?" Before I could answer, he lifted the surgical cap off the troll and saw that it had hair. Turning to Dr. Barrall he said, "Well, it's definitely not me, David!" Dr. Barrall smiled and left to get my release orders and prescription for pain medication.

Mike arrived beaming with joy. He thanked Dr. Herman for all he had done. I got dressed while Mike carried down several gifts and bundles of flowers. Dr. Barrall gave me my instructions and I thanked him again. I checked in with Donna and expressed my hope that we could get together sometime once we both got back on track with our lives. Intuitvely, I felt that we were to become friends through our sharing.

I looked around the hospital, feeling strong and healthy and was reminded of Helen Keller's words, "Although the world is full of suffering, it is also full of the overcoming of it." How true these words rang to me. I had just been given the strength to climb a very difficult, high mountain and I beamed with pride and a sense of accomplishment.

The various shifts and detours we experience on our paths play an important role in our personal development, and what we eventually contribute to the world. We find our purpose by living through these experiences and learning the lessons they bring. Learning the lesson from a difficult experience requires a mental and physical discipline. We must remain still and quiet within ourselves to draw in and absorb all of the lesson being given.

For me this meant facing my troubled emotions revolving around *my* mother and our relationship. By facing this problem within myself, I had the opportunity to break the chain, and not pass this lack of fulfillment on to my daughters.

All the way home I thought about my star I had seen in the corner of our bedroom window. Would I see her tonight? I missed not being able to look outside my window and catch a glimpse of her reassuring sparkle. Something told me that she was right there with me at that very moment. Her presence was warm and understanding.

"Down how many roads among the stars must man propel himself in search of the final secret? The journey is difficult, immense, at times impossible, yet that will not deter some of us from attempting it...we have joined the caravan, you might say, at a certain point; we will travel as far as we can, but we cannot in one lifetime see all that we would like to see or to learn all that we hunger to know."

—Loren Eiseley

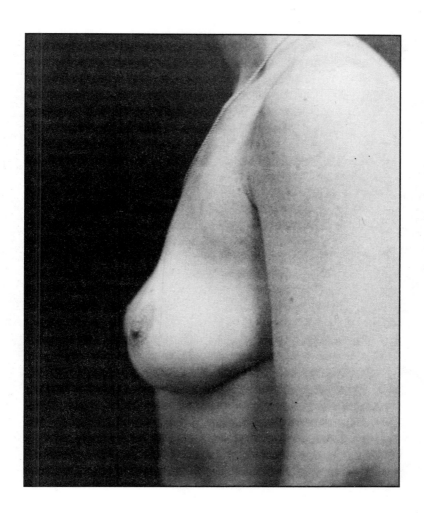

Pre-surgery

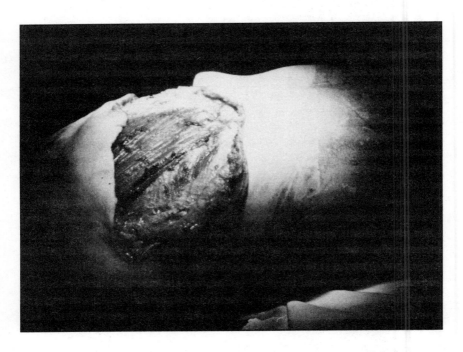

During surgery—before insertion of implants. It was seeing this picture and looking at it repeatedly that truly reinforced my strong belief that a woman is a woman, not through body parts—but, through her soul.

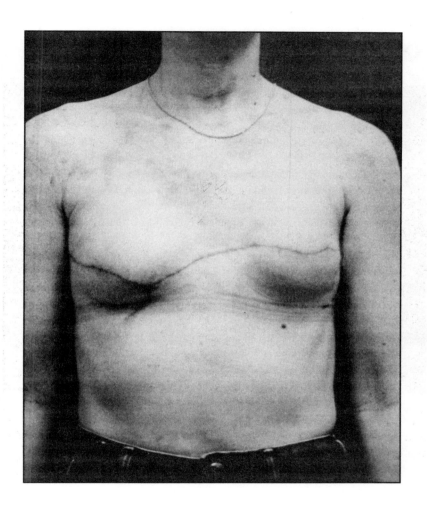

Seven days after surgery.

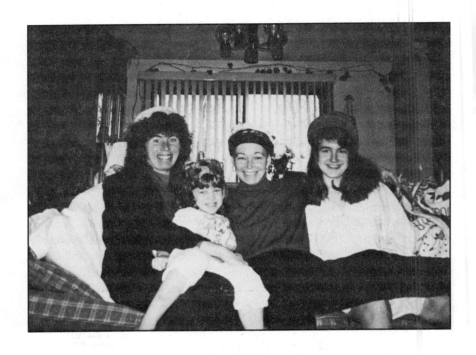

Hat day! Left-to-right: My angel Beth, Meg, me, and Cara

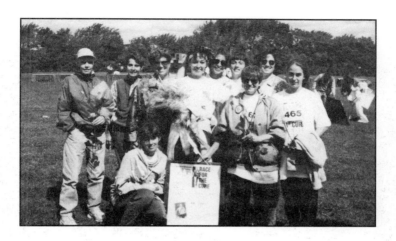

First Annual "Race for the Cure."
Winner of the survivor division!

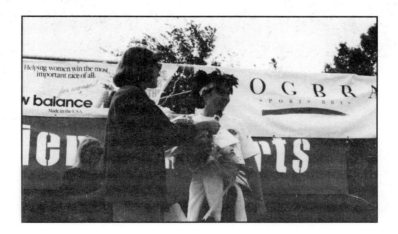

I won! Oh my!

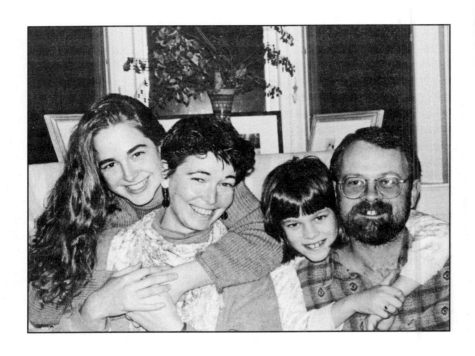

Meghan, me, Cara and Mike.

CHAPTER 7

COMBINING THE EAST AND THE WEST

Jeff and I looked at each other in disbelief. Was I really going home? I had resigned myself to at least five days in the hospital. Being in my own home surrounded by my family felt wonderful and healing. The ride home resembled my ride to the hospital in labor with Cara. My brother, Jeff, had driven me and managed to find every bump in the road. I suggested maybe Mike was putting my new implants through the "American Tourister" challenge to see if they would shake and shimmy like the old ones. He just laughed, but said it was a unique thought.

"These are the new and improved models, so you can quit with your testing strategies." We laughed. I wondered if they would bounce?! I doubt it. Boy, won't it be great to run now. No more pain, and better yet, no more expensive bras.

The house was empty. Meg was across the street at our neighbor's house playing with her friend, Staci. Cara was at soccer practice. I felt deprived missing her practice. We never missed a game or a practice. We shout, yell encouragement and drive the opposing team mad. I knew that soccer would be a great outlet for her. God knows, there are plenty of times when I would love to kick something around to let out my frustrations.

I sat down to breathe in the reality of being home. Steve and Lyn arrived with their beautiful son, Steven. She brought two tantalizing pizzas. Of course, anything looked tantalizing after hospital food. Lyn held out a present, "Here Linda, I bought you a little something that made me think of you." How wonderful, a little purple box stuffed with purple tissue. Inside was a stunning vintage glass pin, with matching earrings, purple of course! Lyn and I shared the same taste for the old in clothes, jewelry, and furniture. Mike fears the rare days that we get together to go antiqueing.

I apologized, "Steve, I could sure use one of those sensational hugs, but I'm afraid my drains will get in the way."

"That's all right, Linda. We'll have plenty of time to make up for lost hugs." We spent a bit of time discussing what lay ahead for me, my family and loved ones. We all agreed that the love and support would be pouring in endless abundance. They made the visit brief, knowing that I needed some rest.

The anesthesia will probably take some time to clear out of my system. My sister, Rosemary, recommended a colonic—similar to a high enema but much more thorough. Unfortunately, the United States does not have many places to go for this treatment. In Canada, and Europe, colonics are considered an important adjunct in health maintenance. Rosemary works as a colonic therapist in Canada, where they see a lot of patients being treated for serious illnesses like cancer.

A few days after a chemotherapy treatment, patients have a colonic to wash out the chemical residues before the colon reabsorbs these toxins. It all made perfect sense to me. When I refer back to some older medical texts, I find colonic therapy frequently mentioned in conjunction with other therapies for treating this illness. Mike had offered to bring the garden hose up and hook it up to the sink. What a smart-ass! He loves to tease my sister, but I'm certain he has the utmost respect for her, and she for him.

Meg came trotting across the street just as Lyn and Steve were getting in their car. She had baby blue eye shadow smudged from her eyelid to the top of her forehead! Steve and Lyn couldn't stop laughing. She looked up at them and batted her lashes saying, "Don't I look beautiful?" Meg gave them each a kiss, and they pulled out of the driveway laughing.

She didn't seem too excited about my being home. I had been so worried about her, and her reaction to her Mommy going through surgery, but she seems fine. It is so true, children have a way of living that we lose sight of somewhere in our efforts to grow up and be "mature." They do creative things just for the sake of pure enjoyment. They need no other explanation. How many of us would plaster on a ridiculous amount of makeup, and trot around town for the sheer fun of it. It would be fun, although it would probably get us committed to the nearest psychiatric hospital. Being inside their minds would be a trip. Their creativity must be similar to meditation for us. Children hook up to the flow of creative energy and go wherever they desired.

I was also certain that children go to their place of peace and higher consciousness. Their minds are free from the pollution of living. They are such spiritual little creatures. I remember reading an article about a family bringing a new baby home from the hospital. Their four-year-old daughter exhibited very hostile behavior towards her new little brother. Needless to say, they were careful not to leave her alone with him.

One day, the little girl asked to be alone with her brother for a few minutes. You could imagine the horrible thoughts going through her parents' minds. But, after the little girl had repeatedly nagged her parents, they asked their pediatrician for advice. He recommended that they fulfill the girl's request, and let her be in the room alone with him. They could stand right outside the door and listen, just in case she did something. The next time the girl made her request, the parents obliged her and left the room but stayed very close to the door. Then they heard the words, "Quick, tell me about God, I seem to be forgetting."

I decided to take a nap, but when that failed, I meditated. Meditation seems to have come a long way since the hippie days. Now, it's frequently recommended to patients for ailments ranging from insomnia to cancer. I have practiced it since my college days although for several years I was unfaithful to a daily commitment. This too shall change.

Rosemary had sent me one of the simplest and most sensible books on meditation. It was titled *Meditation: An Eight-Point Program,* by Eknath Easwaran, a very special and spiritual man. In his book he refers to meditation as a "common sense direction for an uncommon life." He believes that meditation is a technique for training the mind, especially attention and will. He believes that in meditation we are able to set forth from the surface level of life, as we know it, and journey into the very depths of consciousness. He taught meditation for more than twenty years and in 1960, founded the Blue Mountain Center of Meditation.

*"Catch hold of a peace deep within and push it into the cells
of the body. With the peace will come back the health."*

—The Mother
Pondicherry, India

With no concept of time, I brought myself to a place of peace. I was searching for a visualization that depicted health and life. I began to see my physical body as a river. We seldom thought of the river as constantly changing, but it was. New water was brought in, the sand shifted millions of times in the course of a day. These changes represented a constant self-renewal by the river. This is my body, a river always flowing and renewing itself. The cells floating through my body are like perfect snowflakes, so intricate and airy. All the old and less-than-perfect cells gently fall into the flowing river, where they are carried away. Irises bloomed freely along side the river, and the wolf kept a watchful eye. I was refreshed and rejuvenated.

Cara's voice found me and was like music to my ears. I jumped out of bed to greet her, for some reason expecting the same excitement in return. Quickly I had to change my approach. I remembered when my mother first appeared after her surgery. I was so young, and somehow I felt she was a different person. Yes, indeed she was different as I was now. Parts of the difference were visible and other parts were not. My mother hid all of the visible changes that had taken place.

I have grown to be quite the opposite of my mother. It is not uncommon for me to run around the house bareassed after my bath. My children are used to seeing me and I, them. I could offer this important visual connection to Cara now, or I could wait and watch her curiosity and fear eat her up inside. I pulled her into the bathroom. I began unbuttoning my shirt, looking at the same fixated eyes that I possessed 17 years ago. She didn't speak, or make any effort to leave the room. "I don't know if this is the right approach Cara, but I can't bear the thought of you being left out of this, and all I can remember is the pain I experienced when my mother chose to keep it all inside. It was awful, and I never want you to feel that."

"Here," I said as I began unbuttoning my shirt, "feel the new addition to my body!"

She slowly extended her hand, and ever so gently placed it on my chest saying, "Gee, they're awful firm!"

"Yeah, it's going to take some getting used to. Out with the old and in with the new." I chuckled.

"Ya know, every girl should be able to select their own breast size!" We both laughed. She had the well-endowed bust of a Phelan female, which many girls would have killed for. But, perhaps, because she was so athletic, Cara considered them a nuisance.

Meg must have felt the vibes that something was going on, and she was not invited. Invited or not, she made her appearance in the bathroom. She asked in her sweet little munchkin voice, "What are these little balls?" referring to my drains. I planned to explain what they were and their purpose, but instead said, "These little things are my magic balls." She smiled. "They pump in magic healing air so that the boo-boo heals well."

She looked at my chest, "Where are the pink things? You know the, the, the... "

"Nipples?"

"Yes."

I said, "Well they had to take those off."

"That's OK Mommy, because new ones will grow soon." Oh my God, where did she come from? She was not aware that my breasts had been removed. She just thought that these were the same breasts, and they were smaller because they had removed the "bad tissue" from them. I decided to keep it this way, knowing that the truth would only confuse and possibly frighten her. Besides, she had come to this conclusion herself and I didn't feel I had the right to insult her intelligence.

I emptied my magical balls on Sunday and found a minimal amount of fluid in each one. Such a minimal amount, that I wanted them out on Monday. I thought I'd call Dr. Barrall to see what he thought. The poor man was sure to retire if he encountered another patient like me in the near future. I phoned Cheryl at Dr. Barrall's office to tell her that there was really no great amount of fluid in the drains. She agreed to speak to Dr. Barrall. Almost immediately, she phoned me back and said that I could come at one o'clock that afternoon. I would be free from these ornaments hanging from me! I felt like a Christmas tree that had failed somehow.

I phoned Mike and he wanted to drive me to the doctor's. I told him I would have no trouble driving.

"You're not supposed to be driving yet."

"And I was supposed to be in the hospital for six days, too!" I prepared myself a tuna fish lunch in celebration of drain removal. Andrea arrived just in time to accompany me to Providence, insisting that she drive. I didn't have the heart to argue. I was happy just to have her company.

At the office, Cheryl checked out her boss's handiwork and remarked how terrific it looked. It never dawned on me to ask about the procedure for drain removal, but Cheryl explained that the drains were flat and wider than the tubing coming out. One was under the prosthesis, and the other went up into my armpit where the nodes had been removed. Dr. Barrall started to slide them out. Ouch! Cheryl offered me her hand. Resisting the temptation to be brave and macho, I grabbed her hand and squeezed it like an orange.

When it was all over I felt like a free new woman...new breasts and no more drains! We set an appointment for Friday so Cheryl could remove the exterior sutures. Dr. Barrall planned to follow my progress for about a year.

Energy began to fill my body again. I didn't hesitate to reach for my favorite mug, or water the high plants. Sure it felt tight, but I might as well begin healthy, beneficial activity to loosen up the area. My range of motion was surprisingly good. Being in good physical condition at the start had helped. I was not sure how long it would be until I could resume my work, especially the deep tissue work for patients. I would begin with my MLD patients and work from there. Maybe next week? If the doctors only knew...

I spent two hours contemplating whether or not to phone Dr. Herman's office to check on the lymph node report. It had been one week, and I was hopeful. I phoned and Pat said she expected Dr. Herman to check in at any moment. He was at the hospital, the perfect place to check the report. She phoned me back sounding like she was about to burst with excitement. Unfortunately she had only read the first part of the report. After all, it isn't terribly common for patients to have bilateral mastectomies.

She read me the information. "The seven nodes taken from the left were all negative for cancer." Hurray! In the nine nodes taken from the right, one was positive for cancer. It was microscopic, but positive. This still gives me the same prognosis as a patient with negative nodes, or so they say. Zero to three positive nodes share the same prognosis as when all the nodes are negative. How ridiculous. I was regarding myself as a statistic.

I would spit at anyone else who referred to me as just another statistic and here I was doing it.

Mike was already on his way home, so there was no sense in trying to phone him. As he walked in the door, he saw me sitting near the phone and his heart seemed to skip a few beats. I shrugged, "There is one positive f___ing node." I was so disappointed. He tried to comfort me, "Linda, you know darn well that isn't an accurate way of telling whether or not the cancer has had time to spread."

This was not the thing to say. There was not an ounce of comfort in his words. He looked up the definition of statistics. It says "a collection of numerical data." I understood that a doctor was trained to use this terminology, but to me it was terribly insulting. Doctors became doctors to share their knowledge and help others. What was not taught was how to interact with your patients on a personal level rather than a medical level. Fortunately, I found some doctors who just came by this interaction naturally.

Immediately I phoned Dr. Strair. She, too, had seen the report. Her recommendation would be the aggressive CAF. I tried to weasel out of that one by reciting all of the much researched and much misunderstood statistical lingo. She didn't budge. My case was not something you would have seen in a medical text when reading about breast cancer. My family history put me into a zone of my own. Her decision was justified.

I had to decide whether or not I wanted to subject myself to this aggressive form of treatment. In short, I would be asking my body to endure chemical warfare. But, with the understood intention, it would accomplish all that was needed. Another major decision to make. My star shone brightly that night. In such a way, that I knew my star was endorsing what I already felt in my heart. I would do the CAF. Of course, I would be in control at all times, and I could stop if I chose.

Mike was hoping that I would subject myself to this most radical form of treatment. He honestly felt in his heart that it would be the cure. So I closed my eyes and prayed that all I was feeling was right. I began to cry, but not a cry of self pity, rather a cry of accomplishment and relief. I had made another decision.

Thanksgiving was tomorrow, and I had decided to prepare the meal myself. After all, it is my favorite meal of the year. We all held hands in thanks for each other and all we possess. We were blessed with life. It was a beautiful day. I was thankful I had come so far on my long journey seeking health.

Friday morning, I arrived at Dr. Barrall's office for the suture removal. Cheryl had the privilege. The sensation in the incision area was still very numb. I had some sort of sensation in every other affected area. Even my underarms were not numb. It was a strange feeling—like touching your foot when it's asleep. All of the skin covering the prosthesis also had sensation. The strangest feeling was in both sides of my back on the lateral part of my scapula. It didn't feel good to be touched there. I really couldn't explain it...I think the nerves were probably severed in surgery.

I could see that the widest part of the scar would certainly be on my chest across the sternum. Probably because it was resting directly on the bone and was more difficult to pull together. Other than that, it all looked terrific. In a year, the scar would be much less noticeable. Of course, it would always be there. I had accepted this, knowing it would get easier to look at.

I made an appointment to see the doctor in three months. I suspected he just wanted to see how being bald appealed to me. We could compare the bald breasts to the bald head.

Then, I went on to see Dr. Herman. I was actually beginning to enjoy my appointments with him. I always left his office feeling good. I heard his distinctive footsteps. In he beamed with papers in hand.

"Hello there! I won't tell you how terrific you look since you are sick of hearing it, although, it is true. The pathology has come back and I brought it in to share it with you. The other sights of cancer were smaller, but small does not mean insignificant. The one area of concern is in the axillary area on the right side. We may irradiate that site to be sure we cleaned it all out."

"I am terrified of the CAF that has been recommended. What is your opinion?"

He replied, "Linda, you are a young, healthy and vital woman who has to endure a very unfortunate situation. I say put all the bullets in the gun and give it your best shot now, when it really matters." I knew his was the realistic approach, but I was finding it very difficult to find comfort in anything anyone said.

It seemed unreal to think back to when I was a young girl watching my mother go through chemotherapy and radiation. I remember telling myself that I would never subject myself to that kind of treatment. It proved one thing for sure: it was impossible for anybody to know what they would do in any given situation until that moment came for them. This was true of even the simplest things.

Now, I wanted to live. Most of all, I wanted and needed to give of myself. I thought how much I had to offer the world. All the more reason I needed to utilize fully my present experience. Otherwise, how could I possibly consider sharing it with those around me? We would all lose. I realized just how important every decision I made was. Not only to me, but to all those around me whose life I touched and would touch.

There was one thing I knew for certain...I would always receive guidance as long as my heart remained open. I knew I'd always have my guardian angel because I was always aware of her presence. She has guided me and helped me in times of need. The day that I go to meet my creator, she will carry me away to a peaceful and blessed death...hopefully not for about sixty more years!

My date to begin chemotherapy was only two weeks away. For now, I was preoccupied with Meg. She was being weaned from her seizure medication without full consent from her doctor. We began this process in October and she would be free from all medication beginning Christmas day! Her doctor would have preferred we waited until April, which would mark two years—the standard treatment time. Her recent EEG was normal, and having her blood work done was beginning to be a nightmare.

But, the real reason I chose to begin the weaning was because I knew in my heart it was time. Her doctor never argued with me. He only informed me that if she were to experience any seizure activity again, it would probably mean another two years of this poison. I was surprised and grateful that he never tried to make me feel that I was his inferior or not qualified to make the best decision for my daughter. I greatly respected him.

I realized later that the feeling of inferiority was brought on with our consent. If we never consented to it, we would never experience it. I was not the least bit worried about Meg. She was so excited that she would soon be free from the daily ritual of taking this toxic stuff. We seem to be changing positions. I told her that Mommy was to begin taking medicine that would make her feel sick.

Times like this really put my materialistic life into perspective. I realized that professional status meant little. We insist on seeing ourselves through the eyes of others and wonder why we never feel happy. Often we see ourselves at the mercy of the whole world around us. The whole issue of life can be thought of in terms of how we see or define ourselves. Oprah Winfrey once said "...it isn't until you come to a spiritual understanding of who you are—not necessarily a religious feeling, but deep down, the spirit within—that you can begin to take control." So we have to ask, *can* we take control, or does stuff just *happen*? Where do our limits truly end? Are we just a body that stuff happens to, or are we a spirit, and how much control does our spirit have over our body? I believe that the spirit directs the body to fulfill the mission we came to earth with. Often our body helps us to learn about that mission, so body and spirit work together.

For example, how does the body deal with disease? What is really going on? If our body is the physical expression of our spirit and our body gets sick, then doesn't this say that our spirit is expressing sickness? If we only treat the outside expression of the sickness, or the body, then the spirit may regenerate the sickness from inside.

I don't mean to say that it's a bad deal to have the body expressing the spirit. It's rather a question of how you look at it. The other side of the coin is that if the body is the physical expression of the spirit, then the spirit can also *heal* the body. This means finding peace or "health" of spirit is the most important thing for us to do in life.

The spirit/body connection does *not* mean that there is no place for modern medical techniques. These ideas can all work together. In one sense, you could say that even if you have healed the spirit of its wounds, the body still has the leftover sickness in it and must also be healed. We can use both medicine and spiritual energy to heal.

For example, the medical technique of chemotherapy is aimed at killing the fast growing cancer cells. We also know that normally the body reproduces itself about every three months. Cells die off and new ones are produced. So if we have a disease, why shouldn't we picture all these new healthy cells taking over the deadly ones until the good cells win. This visualization of health is a spiritual technique for healing the body. I feel that it plays a very important role in what happens to us.

Once I asked one of my patients how her mother was doing. I knew she had inoperable bone cancer that was quickly spreading to her vital organs. She replied "Well, she's terminal, you know."

I said "That wasn't my question. She's alive isn't she?" My patient just looked at me, but I really couldn't help myself. I explained how unhealthy it was for both her and her mother to be thinking this way. Terminal. They are sending a message to her mother's body that her mother doesn't want to be alive.

It may be more important for her mother to decide if she really wants to be alive. Maybe her spirit has grown tired from neglect and the cancer is a call for help. Maybe it's her way of getting some much needed attention and care. Her mother is the only one who can find out these things for herself.

I decided to return to work on Monday. I had plenty of paper work to catch up on and I looked forward to seeing my patients. I could treat only the MLD patients, but it felt satisfying just to be there. My patient, Laura, was thrilled and surprised to see me. She had her mastectomy surgery some 20 years ago and had a problem with swelling in her arm. I just knew that I could help her. To see her face gave me hope and strength, and I hoped to be able to return the feeling. Before long we recognized a small but significant reduction in the swelling. I couldn't say who was happier. I left the office with a sense of giving. I thanked God for bringing her to me and allowing me to help her.

Going over the Mount Hope bridge that connects Bristol to Portsmouth, I looked up into the pink and purple sunset and said aloud, "God, am I really doing as I should or only as I think I should?" Strange, but I always felt closer to God when going over that bridge. It seemed to lift me up into the heavens. I asked him for a sign. Not a comforting gesture from my guardian angel, without any insult to my angel, but something directly from my creator. Just then, I witnessed the most uplifting and joyous sight that I ever had the privilege to witness. I was about to turn the corner onto my street when I looked up into the beautiful dark blue sky and saw a shooting star!

It may not sound like much, but for me it was the most spectacular event! It was my sign. My assurance that all has been done as it should. It was such a feeling of joy, not happiness, but joy. Joy is a word that cannot be described...only felt through an open heart. Joy feels like a light that fills me with love, faith and hope. Whereas happiness seems to be more of an atmosphere created usually by one's self. Joy is given to us. It can't be man-made. I can't understand how I managed to stay on the road since my eyes never left that incredible sight. By the time I came back to myself, I realized that the car had come to a stop but I can't remember my foot ever touching the brake.

I flew into the house with my feet off the ground. My family looked at me with concern and confusion. When I told them about the star, they just continued to stare at me. Meg understood. She was happy for me. Everytime the phone rang, I repeated my story. I phoned family and friends.

I was in awe. I never doubted God's listening ear but it still remained a miracle to me. The shooting star was exactly what I needed. I was experiencing *bliss*! I always felt that bliss is a joy you experience when you are on the right path. Even though I had encountered this very difficult journey, I was still experiencing bliss because I had the chosen the right path to take me through it.

CHAPTER 8

THE START OF CHEMICAL WARFARE

I had one last visit with Dr. Strair before my chemotherapy began. She was a slight woman with a bright eyes, dark hair and the same sure-footedness as Dr. Herman—a woman on a mission. She told me the lab reports reported my blood counts as terrific and ready to be attacked. We discussed everything about the drugs of choice and their side effects.

I would be treated on a day-one and day-eight schedule and then be left alone for the remaining two weeks so my blood counts could recover. The blood work would be done every week in Bristol, as I had chosen. I had already established a trusting relationship with the phlebotomist at the Bristol Medical Center She was quite good at hitting the vein.

Dr. Strair would keep a watchful eye on my white cell and platelet counts. White cells are vital in fighting infection, so they can not go below a certain limit. Platelets are essential to blood clotting and they keep us from bleeding to death. If these got too low, the treatment would have to be postponed. I had already set my mind on a completion date when I heard her say those words.

Experiencing nausea was inevitable although no one would comment on the expected severity. I could understand that approach. I would really dread it if they told me that I'd be puking my brains out for five days!

There was no doubt I would lose my hair with the dosage I would be receiving. They put a time on it...ninety percent of people lose it exactly two weeks from the first treatment, and the other ten percent, after. I chose to be in the ten percent range.

The nurse also explained that I should expect at least one treatment postponement due to low blood counts. In fact, she guaranteed this would happen at least once. When the cumulative effect of the chemicals was highest the white cell and platelet counts had a difficult time recuperating.

This was normal and practical way to think, but I thought to myself, what's normal? Certainly, I'm not. My pathology report confirmed that. The nurse was not trying to be cruel, she just didn't want me to set my hopes too high. I knew deep in my heart that this wouldn't happen to me. I would do everything in my power to keep my body healthy and strong to cope with all of this chemical warfare. My medical team didn't need to know this, but I was sure they would be asking when it was all over with.

A few wig shops were recommended, including the gift shop in the main building that sold turbans. I hadn't given my bald head much thought up until now. Hearing it discussed made me realize I was not the wig type. There are many reactions to this issue. Many woman choose to experience this disease with as few visible side effects as possible.

I think it is important not to deny this huge change taking place in my life. If I just want to have the fun of wearing wigs, then why not? If I'm pretending I'm not sick, then I've missed the point. I thought if it is socially acceptable for men to be bald, then, why not women? I would have to give this a bit more thought.

Dr. Strair expressed concern about the amount of physical strength and stamina involved in my work. She recommended that I save any strength for regaining my health and that I limit myself to office work. She wrote me a letter of temporary disability for my insurance company, Of course, I had convinced myself that this wouldn't be necessary. But, I stuck my pride in my pocket and asked her for it anyway, just in case I needed to rest at any time. It was a wise decision, I thought.

The staff informed Mike that he would be responsible for the majority of the cooking for the next six months. He didn't look too thrilled. They explained to him that I would experience an intolerance to the smell of food and that it would probably last through the entire duration of the treatments. Oh joy! Cookbooks would be his bible for the next six months.

The girls will not be too happy to hear this. It was time to purchase stock in the Kraft company.

My treatment, all three drugs, was on Tuesday, and my blood work on Monday, to be sure they had the results before the treatment. This was vitally important in order to mix the drugs accurately. They also used weight as a guide. As we were walking down the stairs to leave the building, I decided to institute some little psychological challenges for myself. "Mike," I said, "I don't ever want you to let me even think twice about taking the elevator to the main floor. I want to know that I will always be capable of taking the stairs."

"Oh," he responded, "what if you are not physically capable of taking the stairs?"

"Well then, you'll just have to let me lean on you, babe."

"You can lean on me anytime, honey!" We gave each other's hand a squeeze as though we had just made a very important pact.

Beth phoned and her voice lightened me up. "I have decided that I would like to be a part of this, Linda. I would like to come out on the weeks of the stronger treatments and do whatever you may need... care for the girls, cook, clean, do massage at the office, whatever."

I was both shocked and thrilled. As selfish as it felt, I accepted her offer with enthusiasm.

My dear friend, Rosie, also had no difficulty in lending support. She had her own three-year battle with chemotherapy and radiation when she was just a teenager for the treatment of Hodgkin's Disease. I first met her as a client. She was treating herself to a massage for her birthday and realized how beneficial it had been for the slight edema she experiences in her arms, due to lymph node removal. She was a great friend to have around and the picture of health, not to mention having a superb sense of humor.

We went home and tried to live as normally as possible for the next week. We picked an evening to sit with Meghan and talk about what her Mommy was going through for the next six months, in five-year-old's terms. "Meg, Mommy's boo-boo has healed very nicely, but the doctors would also like me to have some medicine just to make sure that all the bad tissue is gone. I think I should do it. This medicine is different than any kind you or I have ever had. This medicine is going to make all of my hair fall out and I will be bald, but this does not mean the medicine is bad. It really means that the medicine is extra strong and working hard inside of my body."

Mike and I took a deep breath and studied her face. She burst out into laughter! She immediately ran and picked up one of her newborn baby pictures and said, "You mean you're gonna look like me when I was born?"

"Yes Meg, that's absolutely right!"

"Well, don't worry, Mommy. I will make you some dresses for your head so it won't get cold."

Cara chuckled, "Sinead O'Connor move over!" I thanked God that they had the ability and security to still be able to laugh. I knew that Meg would be announcing this bit of information to everybody she comes in contact with so I'd better prepare myself for the possible repercussions. Blessed are we who can laugh at ourselves for we shall never cease to be amused.

Before the treatment started, I did a lot of riding and enjoyed the closeness I shared with Banded. He's one of the best friends anyone could ever have. Horses always listen and they never say anything you don't want to hear. He knew that his life would be changing too. Although he was accustomed to getting a good workout, he wouldn't object to living the easy life for awhile.

I had also been reading a lot lately and Mike recommended bringing my cassette Walkman to the treatment and some tapes to listen to. I chose Bernie Siegel's taped books since they had come highly recommended. Mike would also bring some reading material. We knew that the whole treatment took about four hours. That actually was a long time to sit there and endure both the atmosphere and the treatment. I repeated over and over again that it would be only temporary. The end would come closer and closer with each passing day. We arrived on schedule. My drugs had already been mixed and we were brought into a room by the nurse who would be administering my chemicals. She was quite pregnant and I knew that I wouldn't have her for long. I didn't want to become too attached to her, only to have to adjust to someone new.

She reviewed everything we'd already been told and explained the anti emetic drugs I would be sent home with. Those were to help with the nausea. Poor Mike was about ready to explode with information. They would be giving me Raglan first through the IV, an anti emetic, and Benadryl to counteract the hyper effect the Reglan would have on my nervous system. It sounded like a vicious circle. Then she would administer the Adriamycin, which would be injected through a needle into the IV, and the same for the 5 FU. The cytoxan would be dripped in intravenously.

She showed me into the room where I climbed into a cozy recliner with a little TV attached. She checked my arm surprised that the veins worked so well after having both breasts removed. Normally they had to use the unaffected arm, but in my case I didn't have one. She chose the right arm. The IV needle-of-choice was larger than a standard hand-inserted IV needle. She explained this was because the Adriamycin was more toxic than most and might strip the veins.

The needle was so wide that I broke out into a sweat when she inserted it. I was afraid to imagine if she didn't hit the vein just right on the first shot and had to do it over again! She was also very careful not to let any of the chemicals contact my skin, especially the adriamycin. It can severely burn the skin. Just imagine what it can do in the veins. The nurse, Mary Ellen, had to be especially cautious since she was expecting.

The treatment began. Immediately I felt the hyper reaction from the Reglan. The Benadryl gave me that terrible feeling of being drowsy and out of control, which I hate. My legs were jumping all over the place. I held onto Mike in order not to come jumping out of the seat. I wouldn't let him leave my side.

Within 20 minutes, I had to use the bathroom. So I staggered and swayed my way to the bathroom with the IV stand in tow. I struggled to unzip my pants trying not to use the arm with the needle in it. With the needle halfway up my arm, I was afraid to bend it and screw everything up. I somehow managed and had nearly endless diarrhea. The drug was certainly going to be eliminated. After wrestling with my pants, I had to call Mike to help me pull them up. How humiliating.

I sat down again, feeling that I had plunged into the bottom of an abyss. My eyes rolled so far into the back of my head that Mike wondered if I was gone. It was like being in labor. I had absolutely no concept of time. I tried listening to a Bernie Siegel tape, but it irritated me. I think it was the tone of the music. It seemed too sympathetic. When the treatment was finally over, I looked down those stairs and thought, "Oh no! How am I going to get down these damn things?" But, we managed just fine.

When we got home, Mike put me right into bed, just like a sick child.

He handed me the anti emetic medication. I took it and tried to go to sleep. It seemed like just minutes passed before I bolted to the toilet. I had never in my life experienced such severity of vomiting. I thought I was going to puke out my innards at any moment.

Mike was by my side every minute, prepared to help in any way he could. I began to cry, so helplessly. He brought me back to bed and had set up my large metal mixing bowl with paper towels for puking. Cold face cloths were right next to it and a nice soft towel. It seemed my head was in the bowl more than out of it.

To make matters even worse, our Doberman, Kai, was laying as close to the bed as he could, gagging and puking with me. I thought it was a fluke...maybe he had eaten something that upset his stomach. Between Mike emptying the puke bowl and scrubbing the carpet after the dog, he had a memorable night. I couldn't understand why he just didn't just remove the dog from the room.

Morning—I thought it would never arrive. I could hear Mike getting the girls off to school. He wouldn't let them come in and see me, at my request. By the time they were due home, I would be ready to see them. Once they were gone, I asked Mike to run me a bubble bath. Very rarely did I leave the tub with a problem left in my mind. If I encountered something too difficult to resolve, I always let it go down the drain with the bubbles. I thought it might be soothing this morning. He gladly ran the tub.

I was so weak that he practically carried me to the bathroom. His stare fixed on my abdomen. When I looked down I gasped. It was so indented it looked like there weren't any guts left. He settled me into the warm tub—the keyword being 'warm'. A wave of hot flashes swept over my brain and, within seconds, I was out with my head in the toilet, shaking all over. I sobbed hysterically, begging, "Please don't make me go back. I couldn't possibly endure another treatment. Not without dying."

Poor Mike was terribly humbled by this experience. Our love was so great and this love was all I had at that moment. I looked into the toilet and all I saw was bile. I was puking things from the very depths of my gut up into the toilet. With Mike's help, I staggered back to bed.

I noticed a miniature green-haired troll sitting up on my shelf. I had no idea where it came from or even if I was really seeing it. Mike said he had put it there as a trophy for me. He created his own little chemotherapy head games. I was to receive a new troll after each session. It was so sweet of him. He said Meg saw him with it last night and thought my bride and groom were beginning to start a family. How cute! I lay in bed, begging to be lifted up to the higher more peaceful places and float among the clouds surrounded by health.

Mike had filled the room with beautiful irises and put on some of my favorite Indian flute music. He tried so hard to make it more bearable. "Can I do anything, or get you anything?" he asked in a helpless voice.

I felt I should bring a smile to his face, so I said, "Do you think you could find some cute little fishy decals for the toilet so I don't feel so all alone in there?" He laughed. I must have seemed to be coming back to him.

I finally began sitting up with a minimal amount of vomiting. I tried to meditate and do my visualization. It seemed that all the drugs in my body made it easy to remove myself from the moment. I saw myself galloping bareback on Banded through endless fields of wild flowers. I could feel his immense strength beneath me. He was empowering me. I felt as though he had put himself there in my mind and was willingly giving me his strength. He chose to be there for me.

Mike was standing above me for probably quite some time with a puzzled look on his usually somber face. I was grinning while galloping through the flowers. I opened my eyes and he handed me my anti emetics. I thought, how useless...are they really doing anything or am I just compounding the drugs in my system? "How's Kai?" I asked.

"I put him outside the room, but he cried endlessly and began pounding his seventy-five-pound body against the door every ten seconds, so I eventually had to give in and allow him to be with you."
Animals are so deeply connected with their masters. My horse was giving me strength and the dog was taking some of my pain.

Mike handed me a letter from Rosemary. She urgently recommended that I give myself colonics throughout the treatments. I felt so incredibly toxic at that point that I began to entertain the idea. I needed some input about when to perform them to get the most benefit. I wondered if I even had a colon left in there after last night. After a few minutes, I had a difficult time reading. It felt like my eyes were swelling. Just another side-effect I thought. I would add the colonics to my list of health maintenance routines that I planned to adhere to, which now included vitamins, carrot juice, enzymes and massage.

Mike helped me to dress before the girls were due home. Out of curiosity, I stepped on the scale. I started out at five foot seven inches and 138 pounds. Now I was still five foot seven inches and a whopping 132 pounds. I wondered if I could bottle this stuff and sell it with a guarantee of a five-pound weight loss in the first 24 hours. I could be wealthy in days. Wealthy or not, sick or not—I was still happy to be alive.

My daughters' eyes brought some sunshine into my heart. They reminded me of all the wonderful things in life. I convinced myself that through all of this, I would show them that life was still joyful even at its worst. I could finally manage sitting without any assistance from Mike, so I asked him to go out and purchase a high enema kit. He looked hesitant— like it wasn't on his list of top ten things to do. I said, "Never mind, honey. I'll be out in no time and I can get it." A look of relief came over him.

That was my first night of fairly uninterrupted sleep, with just a faint sense of nausea. By morning, I was up brushing my teeth. That always makes me feel like a new person. Mike slept on the couch these last two nights, for fear of disturbing my sleep. I told him that it would be more comforting to have him next to me.

Again, he got the girls off to school and helped me get dressed. We drove to the drugstore where I know everybody who works there. They had one kit left and I paid for it without any questions asked. In any case, I was totally prepared to answer any inquires about why I was purchasing it—for Mike's grandmother, of course.

The same day, I made an appointment to see the local Naturopathic doctor in Seekonk, MA. Luckily, he had an appointment available in just a few hours. Mike needed to stay home and make supper for the girls. Cara was lacking in culinary arts skills, so I would have to drive myself. I assured him that I was all right driving. I was anxious to meet this fellow and see if my decisions for holistic treatment were similar to his.

Upon meeting, we introduced ourselves and he reviewed everything I had written down, both about my health and the holistic therapies I had chosen. He reminded me of a comedian who was not all together *there*. He had wild hair and stood about my height. His eyes moved about when he was speaking, as if listening to some secret spirit telling him what to say. He agreed with all my choices. We discussed fresh vegetable juice, especially carrot for its high contents of beta carotene, but I had yet to purchased a juicer. I noticed he had a wonderful, heavy duty juicer on sale in his store. It was on sale for $229.00, which seemed reasonable enough for its quality. "Do you by chance have any other models a little less expensive?" I asked.

"No, this is the only one I sell, but I would be happy to sell it to you at cost, to help you out." Another angel—I was very grateful. So was Mike.

Mike immediately began making fresh, sweet carrot juice. It was the first thing I had swallowed since the treatment and I wasn't sure I could keep it down. I drank it and fell into bed for the night, hoping that my exhaustion would override any nausea that might creep up.

Even though I had been ill from the treatment, I felt that my plans and intentions for restoring my physical harmony were appropriate. All I needed now was to keep my intent clear in my mind. I realized that if the mind was fine tuned, it could conserve much of the energy wasted through negative emotions.

At times, it was very difficult to avoid going around and around in the negative thought patterns that bring up the overwhelming negative emotions. But, by knowing that my intent and will were stronger then any negativity, I could bring myself back to center. Every being has the ability to change and grow, but we must also hold a true intent along with the will to see it through. It can be difficult, but I imagine the bliss that will be experienced when we reach higher places will be worth it. Then, we will rejoice and celebrate.

There still was one appointment I felt I should make. That would be at Dr. Deepak Chopra's Auryevedic Health Center for an evaluation. I have always been fascinated by the Indian approach to health, known as Auryaveda. It focuses on continually keeping the harmony within to prevent creating an environment hospitable to disease. I suppose it could be considered a preventative way of living. It has been known to have helped with a cure when all else failed. There is a lot to it, but the simplest explanation is that there are three main body types. They are Vatta, Pitta and Kapha. We usually consist of all three, with one type being dominant. I am certain that I am a Pitta. The body type is determined primarily through pulse. Each body type has specific recommendations to follow throughout the year, which include how to identify the first subtle signs of falling off center and what to do to restore harmony back to the body, mind and spirit.

As anxious as I was to begin Auryeveda, I decided to wait until the chemotherapy treatments were complete. Until then, I would familiarize myself with all of Dr. Chopra's books. So far, my favorite was *Quantum Healing*. Dr. Chopra was a truly inspiring man and writer. In Auryeveda, meditation was highly recommended to bring the mind to an infinite place, free from disease. I had read enough to see that a fast mind was usually the one to take ill. The slow mind seemed to just maintain. But, the still mind was blissful!

> *"A Human being is part of the whole, called by us "Universe", a part limited in time and space. He experiences himself, his thoughts and feelings as something separated from the rest—a kind of optical delusion of his consciousness. The delusion is a kind of prison for us, restricting us to our personal desires and to affection for a few persons nearest to us. Our task must be to free ourselves from this prison by widening our circle of compassion to embrace all living creatures and the whole of nature in its beauty."*

—Albert Einstein

Lately, when I meditated, I could see the river beginning to flow in different directions. For a while, I found myself almost fighting it, thinking it should forever run in the direction I had first seen. But, then, I realized that the river, too, must be rechanneled...sort of a way to break old habits. I even noticed that, in parts, it had been dammed up. These must have represented the unhealthy ways the river flowed for the past several years. And I saw less snowflakes fall into the river. This, indeed, was a very good sign. The garden was beginning to take on new life.

Mike was right on top of getting the carrot juice down my throat. Karen has been a nightly drinking buddy now for a few weeks. We call it our "carrotail hour." She affectionately assigned Mike the nickname "Mr. Greenjeans." I just laughed, but it seemed an appropriate name for him. He loves gardening, and the land surrounding our home shows it. We were already talking about springtime. The flowers would be blooming, the air would be full of life and the birds would sing. Best of all, my hair would be growing back. "Speaking of hair," Karen asked, "When is yours going to start to leave your head?"

"They claim in exactly two weeks, but, just to spite them, I'm gonna hang onto it for three!"

It was wonderful reading the messages at work from all of my loving patients. Deb kept a journal beginning from the time of my surgery. It gave her a way to express herself and kept me in touch with the office. I was deeply moved. I had no idea just what an impact I was having on her life. She worried too much about the office and messing things up. I told her not to worry. I felt she was not just an employee, but a friend. Friends don't have to be perfect.

The barn was always a place of solitude and healing for me, even if I could only spend a short time there. Like meditation, twenty minutes could last for hours. I just stood in his stall and hugged the huge creature that was my horse until I was too weak to hold on.

Trying to keep my next chemo visit out of my mind required some effort. Even though the treatment was to be much milder, it didn't weigh any less on my mind. Mike decided that he would be in charge of keeping track of the blood counts and anything to do with math. My blood was drawn the day before treatment. It was really amazing what effect a place can have on you through past associations...especially the smell. My eyes suddenly felt terribly heavy when we arrived there. Just as they had when we left for the first treatment.

I weighed in at 132 pounds. This was normal, I was told, but they were still worried about it going too low. I didn't get to meet with Dr. Strair for this appointment. It was a quickie, only to take 20 minutes. I apologized to Mary Ellen for having no social manners during the last treatment. She suggested that I shouldn't have the Reglan anymore. Obviously, it didn't agree with me.

We talked more about the head turbans. Mike and I agreed to go into the gift shop to check them out after this treatment. Mary Ellen seemed confident that I would be up to it. They recommended that I take a Compazine for nausea, just in case. We finished up and scheduled my next appointment for the *big one* in two more weeks.

The woman in the gift shop seemed surprised that I was looking for turbans. She was very helpful and insisted that I model some of the newer styles that had just arrived. They looked like ridiculous little Dutch boy hats. I had to laugh and said, "I am only interested in the plain turbans." I tried a few on and insisted on purchasing one in every color that was available. Mike's face turned fairly white for a moment until he heard they only had five colors. I was satisfied. All the way home, I expressed how grateful I was for not being physically ill after this treatment. It was almost a treat.

We had barely gotten onto the highway when suddenly the window went down. I glanced over at Mike and saw a devilish grin on his face, "I just want to see if your hair can still whip in the wind, or if it will whip right out the window!" What a rat! I had complained about waking up some morning and finding my hair on the pillow. That would be absolutely horrifying, not to mention a mess to clean up. So his brilliant idea was to take me on the highway and build up to a nice cruising speed and just let the wind take it away. No mess! Just when I thought that I had such a wonderful, unselfish and caring husband.

I had already made up my mind that as soon as the signs of falling out appeared, I would shave it off. This made me feel I had some control. The other alternative was helplessness. My recommendation to all women would be to shave it off themselves.

The girls came home shortly after us. I showed Cara the turbans and even modeled them for her. She thought they looked pretty cool, or so she said. She would never hurt my feelings. Meg wanted some of her own.

So, I said, "Heck, I think we should all have them and all be bald, so I don't feel so bad."

This didn't go over too well with the girls. I tried them on repeatedly, but I really hated them. They looked so phony on me. I ripped them off and threw them in my closet like a little rebellious child, swearing that I would never look at them again.

I felt I was in a time of heavy transition. The old ways just didn't suit me anymore. They were ripped from my life very abruptly. I sat in that moment wishing that the new ways would just pop into my life, with no effort on my part. No such luck. It was uncomfortable and even painful at times. I thought of the saying, "If you want the rainbow, you have to walk through some rain." I like rain, but this was more like being caught in a hurricane.

We rounded up Jeff's family for our annual tree-cutting ceremony. They use an artificial tree, so this was a grand occasion for the kids. We arrived at their home and my adorable nephew, Timothy, handed me a lovely card he had made. It had a beautiful picture on the front. It read, "I know you have cancer and I hear cancer is a terrible thing. I hope you will be better. Love, Timmy." I was heartbroken.

I had a nice aunt-to-nephew talk with him. I didn't deny that his grandmother had died from this exact thing. Instead, I explained to him that cancer did not have to mean death. Many people can be healthy again. This took a load off his little shoulders. My niece, Jennifer, acted unaffected by my presence. She internalizes too much, just like her father. I made sure she heard my talk with Timmy.

Uncle Jeff was the designated tree cutter and a good one he was! We brought it home and immediately set it up in the stand. I didn't want to miss a minute of enjoyment. I love having the tree in the center of our house to gaze at. It's a symbol of life and an important thought for the season. The hot chocolate and decorating were doubly enjoyable. Every year, the decorations moved higher and higher up the tree, according to how tall Meghan was. It was really funny to compare pictures from last year. Every time we looked at the tree, we laughed. She couldn't understand why!

I was happy to have the shopping completed. It was a modest Christmas, but that's how Christmas should be. If you've lost the real meaning of Christmas, a devastating situation like death or illness will remind you of this truth. Cards are a wonderful way to express the season. I take great joy in writing them, even to my patients. My favorite card that I received this year was from my sister. It read:

> *There is much, that, while I cannot give you, you can take.*
> *No heaven can come to us unless our hearts find rest in it today,*
> *Take Heaven.*
> *No peace lies in the future which is not hidden in this present instant,*
> *Take Peace.*
> *The gloom of the world is but a shadow; behind it, yet within our reach,*
> *is joy,*
> *Take Joy.*
> *And so, at Christmas time, I greet you, with the prayer that for you,*
> *now and forever, the day breaks and the shadows flee away.*

> —Fra Giovanni   A.D. 1513

CHAPTER 9

SHARING

The spirit of Christmas filled my mind so much that I lost track of time. It had been over two weeks since I began chemotherapy and my hair was still on my head. I noticed that my scalp was a bit sore, but no sign of shedding yet. Meghan would soon be off her Tegretol. Hurray!

Cheryl, from Dr. Barrall's office, called to ask permission to give my phone number to Donna, the woman I met in the hospital. With a sudden twang of guilt, I realized I'd forgotten her. "Of course you can give her my number," I replied. "I would love to hear from her." She phoned me the same day to say she had made it through the surgery with flying colors and was very happy with the reconstruction results. She did have three positive nodes. Chemotherapy was recommended. This frightened her, as it would anyone. She had been to Providence to meet with a few different oncologists, but was not happy with any of them.

Choosing a doctor was such an important issue. Many people stick it out with doctors for whom they had no positive feelings. They hear this doctor is good at what he does. That is all most patients feel they are entitled to. If we were hiring help for our business, hiring someone with a personality that suited ours would be just as important as hiring someone who could do the job well. The same is true about hiring someone to look after our health. In fact, we are interviewing the physician. They will be paid for services rendered to us, so we should not only like them, but feel comfortable with their approach.

Donna knew not to stay with a doctor just because he or she had come recommended. Her search brought her to Boston. I was happy that she seemed confident in her decision and that the thought of traveling did not bother her at all. We made a date to have lunch after the holidays. She, too, was due to lose her hair, so we would meet each other bald. Or, she would meet me bald. I told her that I had no intentions of wearing a wig. She told me she had every intention of wearing one. This should be interesting.

Halfway through week three, I woke up and saw a few strands of hair that belonged on my head on my pillow. The sign. The dreaded sign. I went into the bathroom and began running my fingers through my hair, each time getting a clump full of hair. I tried not to cry. After all, I had known it was going to happen. Meg entered into the bathroom and took one look in the sink, and tears came to her eyes. Cara was the only one who seemed unaffected by the loss. I surely didn't expect Meg to be upset after her laughter at being told about it. I was not at all prepared for Meg's reaction.

I immediately stopped running my fingers through my hair, so Meg would calm down. If it were not for her reaction, I would have continued until there was no hair. Quickly I changed the subject and got them off to school. On the way out, Cara asked, "Does this mean that when you come home tonight, you'll be bald?" I said I didn't know, but it would be happening real soon. I asked her if she wanted me to call before I came home so that she would be prepared. She said she would rather be surprised.

The entire day at work I was in agony trying to decide what to do. The most traumatic part was Meg's reaction. I needed to make light of it for her sake. I phoned Donna Marie, my long time hairdresser, aware that everybody would be having their hair done these next days before Christmas. "Donna, I need your help. My hair is falling out and Meg is upset. I need to do something funny."

"No problem, come in around eight o'clock and I'll squeeze you in, OK?" I was grateful.

I arrived and still had not figured out what to do. There would never be another opportunity to relive this and I wanted to make it memorable.

Donna did her magic. The end result was a virtually shaved head with about an inch left on top to spike and a Christmas tree shaved into the side of my head! Nothing like living out all those impulsive moments you had only dreamed about until now! We even colored the tree in green with eye-shadow. This ought to do it, I told her. We exchanged hugs and I wished her a blessed Christmas.

> *"We must march on with the quiet certitude that what has to be done will be done."*

I drove home, laughing to myself the whole way. It felt great to laugh. I ran through the front door and all eyes were on me. Even Mike had no idea where I had been. "Well Cara, you wanted to be surprised, so here it is!" Meg jumped off the couch and laughed with the sound of delight only children can make! I had succeeded, all was well. I agreed that they could share the coloring time every morning and color the tree any color they chose. Mike was still on the couch in shock!

Cara thought it was so cool, "Can I take you to the mall and show you off?" she asked. Karen refused to believe what I had done, so she came over and saw it with her own eyes. She will forever call me crazy. I planned to keep the "do" until after the holidays; that was, if it lasted. Then I would shave it all off.

Patients, mail people, neighbors and just about everybody I saw commended me on my bravery and sense of humor. I thought bravery had nothing to do with it, but the sense of humor was a must. My real goal was to lighten the load for my girls. Public events provided the most entertainment. We went to dinner one night. The entire restaurant was in an uproar over my head. It was certainly an attention-grabber. Some of the talk was pretty degrading, and some was supportive. I can bet that not one person would have guessed the real reason for this drastic *do*...not a one. It was really frightening to realize how much stock we place on appearances. What we really need to realize is that no matter what our color, sex, or life we choose to live, we are all the same. We are all human.

All the back talk I received did not succeed in bringing me down. Not at that joyous time of the year when love was born and heaven touched the earth. That was truly a test—to see if the spirit was in my heart. I passed if terrible things happen to me and I still looked people in the eye and wished them the joy of the season. My heart was filled with a great sense of love and spirit. I was strengthened by knowing that nobody could take that away from me.

Kevin and I had a lunch date. I had grown so accustomed to the new look that I couldn't even figure out why he looked so shocked. We laughed forever, it seemed. He really wanted me to come over when his kids were home so they could see how funky their Aunt really was.

Kevin asked what I had planned to give Mike for Christmas. I said that I couldn't possibly think of anything good enough for him. He said he could! I asked what he meant and he handed me two floor tickets to the Lakers/Celtics game scheduled for January 17. I could hardly believe my eyes. I knew that Kevin would never in his right mind part with these tickets. Maybe another game, but not this one. The whole act was so thoughtful and caring that I just wanted to cry. All he wanted us to do was to have a great, memorable time. I promised we would.

I felt like a little kid. I was sure that I wouldn't be able to wait until Christmas to give the tickets to Mike. I was just dying to see the look on his face when he saw them. I decided Christmas Eve would be close enough. I shared them with Cara. Even she was excited. Jeff agreed to take the girls overnight to make it even more memorable. I booked a room at the Long Wharf Marriott. It would be a blast!

I worried about Meg because she would be completely off her medication. God forbid, if something was to happen to her and I was over an hour away. I knew how important it was for Mike and I to have some one-on-one time together where I could just be his wife and friend without being a mother. We had talked about planning something for every month after the bad session of chemotherapy, so that I would have it to look forward to. The tickets would be a great start.

We decided to attend Christmas Eve mass this year. Mike was not normally one for church, but it had somehow found a place in his heart these days. I can't imagine why. It was your wonderful, traditional mass with all of the music and candles. I couldn't help but notice the two women behind us, staring at my head. I had practically forgotten about it and rarely took notice of people's reactions anymore—but they were right behind us. I turned and offered them the sign of peace. They just smiled that queer, puzzled smile! I smiled back.

We went home, jumped into our pajamas and cooked up some hot chocolate. My tastebuds were still appreciative. Tradition in our home involved the opening of Aunt Rosie's gifts, so that Saint Nick would have enough room to leave his. We all gathered around and joyously opened our gifts. Once the girls were tucked into their beds, "with visions of sugar plums dancing in their heads," we exchanged our gifts.

Of course, I went first. I handed Mike the shirt box that contained our tickets. As his face twisted into the "oh, another shirt" look, I struggled to keep from cracking up! He finally got to the little envelope and opened it. Then, he just sat there with a fixed stare. I thought, what the hell is the matter with this man? I asked him, "Well, do you like your gift?"

"Are they real?"

"Of course, they're real. Do you really think I would have phony tickets made up and then disappoint you?" Then came the sigh of relief! Mike knew that it was virtually impossible to get tickets for this game. If you somehow succeeded, you'd likely find yourself behind a pole somewhere.

Mike handed me three small boxes. All were from Portobello and were incredible earrings. He thought if I had to be bald then at least I should have the most beautiful earrings...a pair of amethyst, a pair of garnets and a pair of blue topaz. I couldn't have picked out a favorite. They were all so beautiful. I said that I would wear the amethyst pair for the Laker game because their colors are purple and gold. He smiled, taking credit for successfully converting a born and bred Celtic fan. He was almost right, but, of course, I couldn't let him know it.

The girls shared in a morning of true joy. I was thankful that my tastebuds had been spared to enjoy my delicious turkey dinner_and Mike was grateful that he didn't have to prepare it! We were truly blessed with a wonderful life.

It was time for me to prepare for treatment—round number two. I decided that now was the appropriate time to do the shaving. The act of shaving felt weighted with some sort of spiritual value. Maybe I should light a few candles and burn some incense in the bathroom to make it a true ceremony. I had to get Mike's help since I was afraid to touch the back of my head with a razor. It was quite the scene. Me, sitting in a big bubble bath, and Mike shaving my head. We should have taken pictures! I couldn't believe how drafty my bare head felt, especially having my head on the cold pillow. It took some getting used to. Having gotten over my little tantrum, I tried on the turbans. I chose the purple one, my favorite, and placed it on my head. It fell to my eyes. Oh great! I had assumed that they were one-size-fits-all. It turned out that I had a small head. The wisecracks poured in from the peanut gallery on that note...small head, small brains, among many others. I threatened to shave off all my hair in the middle of the night if they didn't behave. I meant it, too!

I knew I had to do something, at least temporarily. I took some of my favorite scarves and sat in front of the mirror for an hour until I devised a decent way of wrapping, braiding and tying them on my head. It was not too bad, but the scarves needed to be longer to look fashionable.

Mike needed to take a ride to K-Mart in the morning so that he could purchase an oil filter wrench to change the oil in my car. I decided that this was the perfect opportunity to experience *bald* in public. The thought was both frightening and exciting. This was my first public appearance. I could handle this, I thought. Bloomingdales, definitely not, but K-Mart should be fine. He went one way and I bravely went the other.

I browsed through the scarves. To my delight, I came across several Indian cotton scarves. They didn't look like much on the rack, but, spread apart, they were very attractive. But, the best part was the size. They were wide enough to cover my head— about six feet long. *Perfect!* I took the seven colors and the two prints they had. They were only $1.99 apiece. Mike was happy because I was happy but wanted to know what we were going to do with the $90.00 worth of turbans. I was sure I could convince the nice woman to take them back. After all, they had never been worn.

That night, we skipped the carrot juice and celebrated my new head at one of our favorite little Italian restaurants in Newport. I put on one of my new scarves for the occasion. We had almost finished a wonderful dinner, when a couple with their 20-or-so-year-old daughter and her boyfriend were seated next to us. It was a very small room with little privacy Right in front of us, the woman asked her husband if my scarf was a fashion statement or if I was sick and had lost my hair.

I was shocked that she had made this statement so callously. I wanted to shout in her face, "Er, wrong, I am in a cult and I go around to various Italian restaurants looking for arrogant, obnoxious assholes to kill and eat." Then, I wanted to run out and cry. Mike kept rubbing my leg to reassure me, even smiling a little, to try to take the edge off. He really wanted me to be strong.

She carried on for about 15 minutes. Finally, her daughter told her to shut up, and, for whatever reason I was wearing it, it looked great. Thank God! How she was so lucky to have a sensible daughter when she herself was the epitome of an ass, I don't know. To repay her insensitivity, I intentionally knocked her fur coat down onto the floor when we left. Mike joked that she had an animal killed in order to wear its hair, and here she was making remarks on my lack of it. We took a nice brisk walk so that our lovely dinner wouldn't end with that memory.

Sunday arrived and I was ready for my date with a colonic. Say no more, Mike said. He packed the girls off, so that I would have peace and quiet for the glorious event. I loaded the pillows up on the bathroom floor and rigged the bag of water up on the shower curtain...another time to take a picture! I brought in a few candles and turned on my Shakti Gawain tape. She has a very soothing voice that was appropriate for the moment. I certainly hoped she wouldn't be insulted that I used her tape during a colonic. It really was a compliment. I used the affirmation "cleanse, energize and heal me" throughout the process.

I certainly felt like the river had washed me clean. I would take some time to get used to administering the colonics to myself, but the results were well worth it. It was reassuring to know that I had flushed the excess toxins out of my body before the new toxins came in. I ended the colonic with a few acidophilus capsules and a large glass of Exceed. I had heard from Rosemary that the irrigation would strip away some of the natural flora in the intestines, so I replaced it with the acidophilus. A colonic could also create an imbalance in your electrolytes, so I used the Exceed which was loaded with electrolytes.

I was eagerly awaiting my meeting with Dr. Strair. Mainly to let her know of my dissatisfaction with the anti emetic drugs. I needed to assert that I was in charge of my body. I could call it quits if I felt it necessary. Our meeting was very pleasant and low-key. She was already aware of the unfavorable side-effects I had experienced. She would order another anti emetic.

My blood counts had responded marvelously well. She seemed quite pleased by this. The estimated dosage was correct, although my reduced weight might alter the next batch of drugs since I'm still weighing in at 132 pounds. I would always have to take the anti emetic drugs at home. At least for the first few days after treatment. Since it proved to be difficult to keep even water down without vomiting, Dr. Strair ordered some suppositories.

Today, I met Diane. She would be my nurse for the remainder of the time. Actually, nobody got just one nurse. If one nurse was busy when I came in, I got another. They all seemed very nice, but it was more comfortable for me to build a communicative relationship with just one person. I would hate to have felt that it was impersonal. I liked Diane. She was very sweet and had a great sense of humor. That was a definite plus around there.

Again, I broke into a sweat during the needle insertion. Diane said, "Linda, I would like you to practice deep breathing when I insert the needle. It will help you through the anxiety part of it." The deep breathing created a much calmer experience. I managed to keep up a decent conversation for much of the treatment, but when the Adria came I decided to use some visualization techniques. The Adria was a very pretty bright red color. It reminded me of Kool-Aid, even though Kool-Aid never makes it into our house. I thought I would start referring to my treatments as Koolaid treatments, instead of chemotherapy treatments. Everyone approved.

In my mind, I kept repeating the words, "I have the power to heal myself," until the end of the treatment when Diane was removing the needle. I thanked her, and we made our appointment for the following week. Mike copied down my blood counts and we proceeded to the stairs. No sweat, I thought. I couldn't believe the difference so far. I felt ill, but nothing compared to the horror show last time.

When we arrived home, we found that Beth had brought some home-made chicken soup. She never comes empty-handed! It looked and smelled so soothing. Mike heated up just a few spoonfuls of broth for me. I sipped it down and went to bed.

At six a.m., I opened my eyes to the glorious morning sun peeking in through the lace curtains. I couldn't believe that I slept through the entire night. I had no recollection of taking my medication. Mike and I were so thrilled. In anticipation of me needing him, Mike didn't sleep a wink. He said "I told you that it would be better." But, I still couldn't believe it.

I felt very ill —I could blow at any minute—but, I was gaining some control over it. I knew that my intent was sincere. I was doing my best not to let any negative thoughts in my mind interfere even in the worst moments. I felt that my inner healing process was beginning to take shape.

The repressed anger from my Mother's early death was finally working its way out with my assistance and acceptance. On this thought, I would like to share with you a paragraph from Carl Jung's *Modern Man in Search of a Soul:*

> *To cherish secrets and restrain emotions are psychic misdemeanors for which nature finally visits us with sickness...It is as if man had an inalienable right to behold all that is dark and imperfect, stupid and guilty in his fellow beings—for such of course are the things that we keep private to protect ourselves. It seems to be a sin in the eyes of nature to hide our insufficiency—just as much as to live entirely on our inferior side. There appears to be a conscience in mankind which severely punishes the man who does not somehow and at some time, whatever cost to his pride, cease to defend and assert himself, and instead confess himself fallible and human. Until he can do this, an impenetrable wall shuts him out from the living experience of feeling himself a man amongst men ..."*

—Carl Jung

This illness has forced me to evaluate my thoughts about death. Most people don't give much thought to death because it scares them. Perfectly natural, I suppose—but shouldn't we think about it? While we may accept that after death we will not be living on this plane anymore, are any of us sure about the level of existence on which we *will* live?

We'll find a much higher plane, I am sure. I believe we will meet with our creator and be born again and again. While death is not yet welcome in my heart, I don't fully fear it. I do fear leaving my children behind...they'll need me. I know in my heart that my work here is not nearly complete. I have a great sense of life and of continuing to live after death, in my spirit. I truly believe I will survive.

It became clear to me why some people find it easier to die than to change or make adjustments. Dying can seem like an easy way out compared to facing your inner self and making the changes that enable you to live. I choose to make my changes or transitions in an accepting manner. I see that I have been given a chance for a more enlightened life. I would never claim that these changes are not difficult, even excruciatingly painful, at times, but they are all part of the process of growth.

I also believe that we have selected our own road for growth prior to reaching it in this life. So we must *experience* our trials and grow through them. There are no shortcuts. The disease we experience is the physical expression of our inner imbalance. If we become unaware or detached from the symptoms of our disease, we will hurt ourselves by denying our chance for growth. For me, it has been a truly humbling experience thus far.

I had prayed not to be ill during our anniversary and my prayers were answered. Our normal celebration with dinner at our favorite restaurant wasn't possible. Instead, we hugged a lot and spent the evening rejoicing in each other. My love-life was not something that I usually discuss, but I feel its an important issue for women who have lost a breast or two. It's true, I'm blessed with a wonderful husband, but, more importantly, I'm blessed with a great measure of self-love. My self-concept helped me present myself to my husband as romantically as I normally would, in or out of bed. Love-making was as wonderful as it had been in the past, if not more so. He was not afraid to touch. I was not afraid to be touched. It was my body, after all, and my beauty was within.

I must add that if it is true that there are leg men, butt men, or breast men—Mike was definitely a breast man. So, I suppose he made all the necessary adjustments to my body and took the time to learn the new shape. I did not have the same sensation in my "breasts," but it was so important to be touched there. I don't believe we should limit ourselves according to this taboo. It would be like me massaging somebody and forgetting one leg. They would certainly notice the difference when they stood up and somehow wouldn't feel whole. I call it "body deprivation." As we lay there in bed, with candles lit all around us, we embraced each other and celebrated another glorious anniversary.

The chemotherapy reaction was beginning to wear off but the flu-like symptoms I'd been experiencing for about a week seemed to be getting worse. I couldn't bring myself to say anything when I had my treatment for fear of postponing it. If my blood levels were fine, then the light was green. I did some paperwork on Thursday, still feeling out of sorts. I was drinking my juice and taking all of my supplements. The game was the next night so I had to shake this, quickly.

Friday came and, by the afternoon, I was shaking with the fever chills.

I was hysterical, haunted by the memory of the doctor telling me that if I became ill with a virus, I would be hospitalized. Of course, that made sense. If my white counts were too low, there would be no internal mechanism to fight the infection. I would have to lay in a hospital and receive antibiotics intravenously. In my mind, the worst part was that the treatments might be delayed.

I couldn't allow any of this to happen. It would be a cold day in Aruba when they could get me into a hospital where I might be exposed to even worse bionic germs! My mind was twisting and turning in so many different directions. I got into bed and sobbed uncontrollably for an hour. I was burning up inside and my hysterical state was not helping me. I took my temperature: 102°. I panicked. The doctor said any temperature over 101° would be grounds for hospitalization. Please, God, don't let this happen.

I called Mike and really freaked him out. I was totally incoherent. I told him that there would be no possible way I could make the trip to Boston. He said, "Big deal, honey...we'll stay home and take care of you." I despised those words, "take care of you." He promised that we would still make next week's game. The best thing to do was to phone Kevin, in case he wanted to use the tickets. He was still at the office, but Mary was home.

It must have startled her to hear my hysterical state. She immediately began to speak in a very calm voice, trying to soothe me. She spoke to me for a long time and I told her everything. She responded, "Linda, its perfectly fine if you have to be in the hospital for a few days. That doesn't mean that you have failed in all you are doing. It just means that you are still trying to control the rest of the universe—while the focus needs to be on you, right now. Being in the hospital will give you time to rest, read, write and be good to yourself." It was encouraging. I was almost agreeing with her.

Mary continued, "Its time you take yourself off your sphere. You need to be you, for you, right now...not a wife, not a mother, not a friend and not a massage therapist. These are all giving positions. Its time for you to be on the receiving end. In order for you to successfully make any long-term changes, you need to look honestly at your life and realize that it is nice to be needed, but not at the expense of your health and sanity."

Oh, God, how I would have given anything to have Mary at my side at that very moment. I was grateful to at least hear her voice—even over the phone. I thanked her. She would have Kevin call me. She tried so hard to find more encouraging words for me. I figured she was afraid to let me off the phone knowing that I was alone. I promised her that I would be fine and that Mike was on his way home. Finally, she allowed me to hang up. I laid my head back on the pillow and wrestled with my anger. I knew Mike was going to insist that I phone Dr. Strair. If I can put him off long enough, maybe she'll have already left the office.

It was three p.m. and the girls were due home any minute. Just as the thought left my mind, the phone rang. It was Mary! She had grabbed a book and found more healing words. I was so grateful. I knew she was really checking up on me to make sure I didn't do anything silly. Of course, this would have never been the case, but I'm sure that hearing me sound this way was worrying her.

Mike came home with that same pathetic look of concern on his face. I felt like a whining, blubbering idiot totally unaware of the negative effects these emotions were having on my body. Get a grip, Linda. I phoned Dr. Strair. She insisted that I get in right away to have my counts done. After she saw the results, she would decide what action was appropriate to take. I half begged for and half insisted on some oral antibiotics and just good old bed rest.

There was no getting out of the blood work. Mike practically carried me to the car. I was still shaking and crying. I'd never met the phlebotomist who was about to stick my veins but we were off to an unpleasant start. She was not too pleased that I came in just when she was leaving. I could barely hold my arm straight. She poked me and nothing happened. This just made me more hysterical. She poked me again— still nothing. This time she just twisted and turned the needle until, finally, she had some blood flowing. She pulled the needle out so fast that blood spurted everywhere.

I wanted to slap her. She was an arrogant little twit with no compassion! My platelet counts were so low that the bleeding took longer than usual to stop. This wasn't a good sign—at least to me, anyway. And the twit seemed to resent having to wait around to make sure I didn't bleed to death. By then, I was so upset and vulnerable that all I could do was sob.

We went home and awaited the decision. My blood counts were not very high but they were acceptable. She ordered a strong antibiotic and I was to phone her tomorrow if I didn't improve. Knowing that I was going to be able to stay home, I immediately calmed down. My temperature quickly dropped to 101.4°. Thank goodness.

Karen came over for our 'carrotail'and was surprised to find I was a basket-case. She had never seen me in this state and I figured she probably would choose never to see it again. She calmed me down a bit more. I insisted that Mike call a friend and go to the game without me. He resisted several times and finally I ordered him to go. He called a friend who eagerly accepted the invitation. Karen offered to stay, but I was already feeling much better. The girls would take care of me.

Kevin was concerned, but happy that Mike was using the tickets, too. He needed to get some distance for a while. Off they went...and off I went to the tub—fever or no fever!

Snow was falling when I lay down...a very beautiful snow, light and airy. I lay on the bed and stared up into the sky where my star usually was. Reading a few pages from Eknath's book, I came across how he compares the mind with that of an elephant trunk. He says;

> *"The mind never rests....it goes here, there, ceaselessly moving through sensations, images, thoughts, hopes, regrets, impulses. Occasionally it does solve a problem, or make necessary plans, but most of the time it wanders at large, simply because we do not know how to keep it quiet or profitably engaged."*

I can understand this now that I have seen and felt the destruction from this pattern of behavior. The ceaseless wanderings of *my* mind had been repeating patterns of control. Looking back on my reaction that night, I realized how right Mary had been. This experience mirrored my inner imbalance. I had shut down the flow of life with overcontrol. By trying to control everyone's lives, I had hoped to make up for the pain and loss of my Mother's death. I saw myself as—*in there*—making sure it all went well for them and preventing their hearts from experiencing the same lack mine had.

Of course, I had taken on an impossible task. My efforts to control every situation worked against the growth and love I wanted to experience and share. It took a disease within a disease, like this small case of flu, to get me to let go. Letting go, I was able to receive the comfort and care that I needed to get really well. I realized now, it was safe to turn off my controlling mind and let God have the reins. So I lay there in bed repeating my mantra and finding myself begin to settle down. Before I knew it, I was asleep.

Mike was leaning over me, when I awoke, stroking my forehead. I felt fine. He said my head felt cool, no temperature. What a relief. Tomorrow, my blood counts would be done again before my less traumatic treatment. Hopefully, they would be fine. Everyone seemed to have heard about my hysteria and was calling to check up on me. As much as I appreciated their words of concern, I really would have been happier if they hadn't found out about this little incident. I had already chalked it up to just another learning experience.

I called Mary to thank her for being there and lending me her support when I needed it. I'm sure she had been divinely guided to be home for that reason. I think she was a little surprised, "Linda, I knew you would be all right, whatever happened. I knew this because of what happened the day we came to see you in the hospital following your surgery. We were leaving, and just as I walked out the door, a little angel came to me and told me you're going to be fine. It was an incredible experience, but I believed it."

Tears came into my eyes and I felt confirmed in all of my feelings, even about my angel. I knew in my heart that the angel selected Mary because she knew Mary would hear her. Inside, I was filled with joy and hope. I didn't think Mary would ever know just how I felt...but, maybe someday she will.

The blood was drawn and we proceeded to Providence, as scheduled. My blood counts were all right for this treatment. Of course, Mike wrote them all down again. We came home and I crawled into bed, feeling a bit nauseous. I guess I slept for a few hours.

Very little time was spent in the office this week. Beth and I spoke on the phone. Even though she came out to stay during my treatments, I rarely saw her. She was either working or running. I was either puking or sleeping. We promised each other that we would spend some 'quality' friend time somewhere along the line. Two of my support members, Karen and Rosie, seemed to keep their distance. I think it must have been difficult to witness everything I represented right now. It must have hit pretty close to home. Karen was always bringing something over, flowers, etc., but never made it to the bedroom herself. She always gave her gifts to Mike and told him to give me a hug. I certainly don't blame her.

Andrea spends a lot of time with me after a treatment, or at least it seems like a lot of time. The drugs have a tendency to distort time. She came when I was hysterical and she'd come any other time I might need her comfort. She stays connected to my needs and always shows up when I most need the support. I know she will let me cry with her, without judgment, assuring me that her prayers are endless.

The much anticipated game day finally arrived and I was feeling strong. We dropped the girls off and went on to Boston. We ate a terrific Mexican dinner and even managed to throw in a little romance. Come morning, we were as excited as two little kids. The game wasn't due to start until noon, but we decided to try to sneak a peak during practice. We took a taxi to the garden, an experience in itself. We figured the Boston cabbies must teach the New Yorkers how to drive. Well, we made it. Sure enough, they were practicing, all except Magic Johnson—our favorite. He's so good that he doesn't even have to warm up. At least, this was my thought. To watch these magnificent athletes right before us was an incredible experience. They are so tall, yet so graceful.

Here were two nuts from Rhode Island, dressed like L.A. residents. I had a *Magic* sweatshirt on with a purple and gold scarf wrapped on my head and was wearing my amethyst earrings. Mike had his Magic Johnson sneakers, hat and sweatshirt on. Its a wonder we weren't killed right then and there. The most incredible moment happened just at the beginning of the second half. Magic was standing ten feet in front of me when he turned around and looked right at me and Mike in our groupie getups. He gave me the most beautiful smile...you know the beautiful smile I mean. I nearly jumped out onto the floor to hug him. What an exhilarating feeling! Better than eating a peppermint patty from atop a mountain, with the wind whipping through my hair. For those brief, wonderful moments I was not a cancer patient. I was just Linda, having a great time and feeling wonderful. That was a memorable weekend.

The game ended. The Lakers dusted the floor with the Celtics. I was happy about it. Of course, Mike was doubly elated, walking out of the Garden with that proud look planted firmly on his face. As we left, an elderly couple seated in front of us on the floor turned and wished us a nice visit in Boston, assuming we were from L.A. When I told them that we were from Rhode Island, the woman looked like she was going to spit on me! Oh well, you can't deny a good team when you see one.

We talked about the game all the way home. I asked Mike, "What could we possibly do next month that could match this?"

"We could always fly to L.A. and see a game!"

"Another year, honey, when I have hair." On the way home, we planned a good diversion for after the next treatment. We decided that it would be nice for me to see my sister, Rosemary, just for three days or so. She had not been able to come out here. That was all right. I knew she was with me in spirit...only a phone-call away. The change of scenery would do me good.

I phoned Rosemary to see if it would be all right. She was thrilled. The reservations were for Valentines day. I would be halfway through my treatments, a time to celebrate. I asked her to bring Janie, a mutual friend, with her to pick me up. We would go to my favorite Chinese restaurant in Toronto—*Yong Loks*. She thought that sounded peachy-keen! It was settled. I would see her next month. Since my birthday was on the twenty-first, it would be a nice present. She would plan a visit to Rhode Island in July when all of my treatments were completed.

I meditated more than usual. I felt every extra minute my mind was away from disease and treatments was an extra minute towards health and well-being. To transcend this plane in meditation was a profound experience. It gave my body, mind and spirit a chance to realign themselves. The river continued to flow—making new and healthier pathways.

"Forward forever forward. At the end of the tunnel is the light...
at the end of the light is the victory!"

—The Mother
Pondicherry, India

Not much thought has gone into turning 30. Age was not significant to me. This attitude probably rubbed off on me from my mother. My Aunt Marge claimed that all Phelans aged like a good wine...getting better with every year. She was referring to our physical bodies. I hoped that it would reflect on my *life* with the same meaning. I wanted to live my life like a spider weaving a beautiful web, so when I stood back, I would see all its woven beauty.

Work was even more meaningful those days. I began to see the people in my life in a different light. Before my illness, I saw my clients as *just clients*. Now, I realized that everyone in my life was there to somehow share my path. Some people seem terribly familiar to me. When we meet, I'm sure that I already know them. For others, it takes longer before their purpose in my life is revealed to me.

The type of body work that I do makes me especially susceptible to sharing energy with my clients. I realized that my clients were there in my life to benefit me as much as I was there to benefit them. These exchanges were part of the special gifts of the universe. I was thankful when everyday I could go to bed and know that I had contributed to the love and nurturing in our world.

Mike took the girls to the movies so that I could have my Sunday colonic treatment in privacy. I set the bathroom up, shut off the phone and listened to some Indian flute music. I'd actually begun to look forward to these treatments knowing how much better I would be feeling. In the middle of the treatment, I broke out in a sweat. This was due to releasing some toxins. Rosemary had already explained the process to me, so I was prepared for this reaction. I soaked in a nice hot bath, afterwards, and felt like a queen.

It was equally important for Mike to have some time away with the girls. Cara always came in and teased me a little bit about stuffing a hose up my rump. I told her to watch out because I just might decide to stick it up hers, someday. She asked what army was going to help? I assured her that the day would never come when I needed help! We both chuckled.

Chemotherapy treatment number-three was just about here. I wondered what to expect from this one. I had experienced the after-effects of both extremes and this made me a bit edgy. But, the glass was going to be half-full soon. Then, I would have a wonderful trip to Canada, followed by my birthday. It would be a busy month.

Beth arrived and the office was in order. My blood work was done and we took our usual trip to Providence. I wondered if I would ever be able to make the trip to Providence again without getting nauseous. The mind is such a powerful tool. The smell of the building began to nauseate me. I wished I could be home for the actual treatments. I brought Vicks and hard candies to suck on during the treatment. It was the strangest feeling. When the Kool-Aid entered my veins, it rushed to my head and I could smell and taste it. It tasted weird and not very appetizing.

Again, my blood counts were very obedient. I thought, that's my blood—tough as heck and ready for anything. I was proud to have such wonderful blood. It was a few moments before Diane came. In the meantime, a new nurse administered a treatment. She asked how I was feeling. I said I was hopeful and grateful that I would soon be halfway through it.

"Oh no," the nurse said, "this is the worst time. People look at all they have endured so far and realize that they have the same distance to go. Suddenly, being halfway through doesn't look so good." I thought, the nerve of this nurse trying to bust my bubble! I was *still* half-full. Diane came in all smiles, as usual. No misses with the needle, but the same old sweats. She asked if I was experiencing difficulty sleeping, or any leg cramping.

"No, thankfully." Now, I knew to expect these symptoms—like the ulcers that I was to get in my mouth. But, nothing, so far...not as long as I could help it. I had recently purchased a lavender Irish cap to wear. Diane just loved it. So did I. I loved hats. This one made me feel special. The treatment went well, as did my visualization, and the stairs were no problem. I was all set until next week. Then, I would be on my vacation!

We made it home. Mike insisted on doing everything the same way we had last time, hoping to have the same outcome. No such luck. I was up and in the toilet within two hours, crying again. But, that stopped. I took control of myself this time. Crying was becoming a pathetic cop-out and I would not allow it to interfere with my will. He eventually brought in the dependable puke bowl. As usual, the dog was as tightly squashed next to the bed as he possibly could be.

I felt more delirious from this treatment than I had with any others. I thought it must have been the cumulative effect. I kept forgetting the bowl was next to me and, instead, kept dashing off like a drunken sailor to the toilet. I was collecting myself and washing my face when I saw the fishy decals in the toilet. I couldn't laugh, but I was a bit bewildered. Were they for real and, if so, where on earth did he find them? Well, that wasn't important, but they sure as heck were cute.

By morning, I was still ill. That really put the pressure on Mike. I said, "Please, just take care of the girls, you don't need to be in here every minute cleaning this damn puke bowl." Once the girls were off, I asked, "So, where did the fish swim in from?"

He chuckled, "Never mind, I just hope they help."

While I recovered, I thought about what a dynamo of energy I had been before the chemotherapy. Imagine what all that energy could do when directed in the right paths? Instead of depleting myself by racing off in different directions trying to be the perfect wife, mother and therapist, I could be focusing on my inner growth. Before now, it never occurred to me to use my energy to achieve what *I* needed on *my* path. Set limits—I could not—because it was impossible to have limits on oneself when there were no limits on the unknown. This was somehow comforting. I was very peaceful for many reasons.

My first conclusion about my new found peace was that I had accepted my circumstances and all my decisions that went with it. I found that peace comes from acceptance, and freedom from forgiveness. It was easy to think that I had forgiven someone for something they may have done or said, but my words had to be felt through my heart...then, I was free. I spent many hours reflecting on my life and many times I thought I had forgiven someone for something very painful. When I went back and found that the issues were still as painful as the day they had happened, I realized that true forgiveness had not taken place. I was never free. The pain kept me tied to that person and the negative energy associated with them.

Beth came out late that week so that she could spend the weekend with me and take me for my treatment on Monday. It relieved Mike for the day. I think she needed to see and experience this with me for her own reasons. I felt better when she said that the smell irritated her too. She could tell by my face that I was not feeling as well as I had after the smaller treatments. She brought me home and made sure I took my medication. Once I was in bed, she went home. I lay in bed and realized that in a few more days I would be visiting with my sister in Canada!

Jeff took me to the airport. I looked forward to getting on that plane, but I knew the tug felt from home would be strong. I did need to do this for myself. Sitting in front of me on the plane was a woman and her seven-year-old daughter. She asked her mother, "Why does that lady have a scarf on her head?" Her mom replied, "Well honey, she may be sick and on medicine that makes her hair fall off, so she wears a scarf on it to keep it warm." This seemed to satisfy her for now.

It was about five o'clock in the evening and the sun was beginning to set. The colors were spectacular. We took off into the beautiful sky and once we were above the clouds, I looked out the window. I felt like I had just entered the gates of heaven. I couldn't remember ever seeing such a wondrous sight before while flying, and I had certainly spent many hours in airplanes with my mother. I thought, at any moment, I would see a little angel sitting on one of the pastel color clouds, waving to me as I passed her. It was truly a magical moment. I have never felt so close to my mother as I did that moment, even when she was living. I felt her spirit surround me and I cried.

The little girl immediately looked at her mother and asked, "Is she crying 'cause she doesn't have any hair?" I told her that I was fine and that being up here in the clouds made me think of my Mommy. She just smiled, a sweet seven-year-old's smile. I missed Meghan already!

I arrived in a blizzard. Rosemary and Janie had been tied up in traffic due to the bad weather but got there shortly after I arrived. We hugged and talked and I could tell Rosemary was relieved to see me looking so healthy. Even my skin was terrific. We porked out at Yong Loks and ordered enough to bring home. We must have stayed up later than I had in four months. We talked and I showed her my scar. We spent some quality time, sister to sister. She realized that the last time we had spent any time alone together was ten years ago...much too long.

It was a wonderful visit, the highlight of which was the little birthday party she threw in my honor! She made the cake as decadent as my strict diet would allow. It was a celebration of the day I joined the earth, the sky and the people. It was a sad departure, but I wanted to see my family. She had stuck a card inside my bag to open on the plane. It was a very personal card and it touched my heart with much love. It was a curious thing...it seemed the more I read from the ink of my sister, written through the love in her heart, the better I knew her and the closer I felt to her.

The ultimate thrill was coming home to my family and finding all was well. I felt another year enlightened. After all, how many woman get to experience their thirtieth birthday while being bald? As if turning thirty isn't memorable enough. But, I must admit, the most incredible gift I received was from my dear, sweet brother, Kevin. He gave me a great pair of tickets to see Steve Winwood in July. Be still, my beating heart!

I was not home for more than an hour when I learned that Donna had been admitted into a Boston hospital. She had the flu and her blood counts had dropped dramatically. For a brief moment, I felt her pain. I immediately phoned her and was relieved to hear her voice. I could tell that her spirits were good. I had to admit she was handling the situation much better than I think I possibly could have. She said "I can't stand this, Linda. I don't think they're going to release me for another three days."

"Worry not, honey. I know the perfect plan. Just drive them crazy and threaten to climb down tied bed sheets if they keep you any longer. The thought of a possible fall and lawsuit will straighten them right out!"

CHAPTER 10

THIRTY AND BALD

My angel, Karen, stopped by with a birthday gift and a card. I couldn't help but notice her excitement. Since it was only the night before my birthday, I knew it had to be special if she couldn't wait a few more hours. Of course, to stay within the realms of etiquette, I had to open the card first. It was an animated card with three hyenas on the cover rolling all around laughing. The caption read, "For your birthday—a joke so funny it is going to make you laugh your boobs off!" And the inside read, "Oh, I see you've already heard it!" I thought I would just die! Only Karen could find a card like this and get away with giving it to me. I looked at the box and was certain that the gift would surely make up for the card in terms of meaning and appropriateness. Not a chance. I opened the box to find an oversized T-shirt which reads, "I'd rather be 30 than bald!" I couldn't wait to pay her back.

With chemotherapy treatment number-four approaching quickly, I read that medical researchers were studying a new protocol for the treatment of breast cancer. The treatment time was four months instead of six. I thought I would just run that little bit of information by Dr. Strair and see what she had to say. Beth was due out as usual. I looked forward to her energy in the house. The drive to Providence was beginning to feel like some sort of perverse self-torture. Thank God, they treat me right away. I was sure I could never hang around in there and just wait.

As usual, my counts were very reliable. My weight was also holding its own. I was anxious to ask Dr. Strair how everything was going. I told her that if I had to taste another mouth full of bile, I would provide her with grounds to commit me. There was not much else for her to do to eliminate the nausea. A Scopolamine patch, worn behind the ear, might have helped a bit. The fact was that I would just have to ride out the remaining treatments with the nausea. The nausea was a fact I chose not to reflect on. There was a new drug called Zofran awaiting approval from the FDA. They found it was very successful in eliminating nausea due to the adriamycin combination. Of course, it was not available to me.

Diane was chipper today. I was determined to keep my heart rate down during the needle insertion so that I wouldn't experience the sweating and the nausea that accompanied it. It tested my ability to separate myself from the physical situation. Oh, how important it was for me to pass this test. I began the visualization with my head...seeing and feeling the warm, golden relaxation pouring through every nook and cranny...slowly working its way down through the rest of my body. I could hear the voices of the people working on me, but not their words. I continually repeated my mantra to myself. Before I knew it, I opened my eyes and found the needle in my arm and taped in place. Both Mike and Diane seemed pleased that I had finally succeeded in mentally surpassing the emotions brought on by the needle.

It felt like there was some sort of a catalyst in my brain. All I had to do was find it and activate it. Then, anything was possible. It was difficult for me to be clear about this. I sensed an inner knowingness. The catalyst was the way to get to that "knowing." I spoke for a while with Diane, going into my quiet time. She said "Linda, I hope that you're not going to be to hard on yourself if you do have to experience a postponement in treatments. This is very aggressive treatment. You should try to be prepared for it. It is a difficult task that your body is trying to accomplish. You must respect it and allow it the time it needs." I smiled and told her that when I tell my counts to jump, they stand to attention and ask, "how high?" We laughed.

We survived treatment once again and made our exit down the stairs. Mike played nanny and tucked me into bed. This was beginning to get old, I thought. Surprisingly enough, this was not a terribly bad night. I was ill, but it didn't seem as severe as the last time. Maybe it was because I am nearing the end. The glass was getting fuller by the minute! I was having difficulty looking at Mike's fish tank without feeling like I should be sticking my head in there and barfing. The decals were amusing but they needed to go. An association was beginning to develop.

I lay in bed with a clear view of my star. The moon was exceptionally bright tonight, so as I lay there I tried to absorb as much of the energy as I could. I began to wonder just how connected I am with this star. Will I ever know?

> *"No theory of physics that deals only with physics will ever explain physics. I believe that as we go on trying to understand the universe, we are, at the same time, trying to understand man. Today I think we are beginning to suspect that man is not a tiny cog that really doesn't make much difference to the running of the huge machine but rather that there is a much more intimate tie between man and the universe then we heretofore suspected...the physical world in some deep sense tied to the human being."*

> —Dr. John A. Wheeler

Day two—I began to feel quite ill. All I really wanted to do was eat a bean burrito. I said "Mike, would you be terribly disappointed if I tried some of the 'wonder weed' (marijuana) that was given to me?"

"Are you crazy! Anything that could help you through this is all right with me. Where is it anyway?"

I had hid it in my underwear drawer, completely unaware that the bag was not sealed tightly. Consequently, all of my underwear smelled like pot. I took out a pipe that a friend gave me and stuffed the pot down into it. I felt like a naughty teenager. I never liked the stuff, but if it worked...who knows? I nearly died trying to inhale.

After a few drags, I lay down, as if expecting this outrageous trip to occur. All I experienced was a dry mouth. That alone was a spectacular result. The extra saliva your mouth produces for some reason seems to be a big factor contributing to the nausea. The paranoia was beginning to set in. At one point, I thought I hadn't put the pipe out all the way because that was all I could smell. I looked in the drawer where Mike had put it, but it was out. Then I worried that Cara would be able to smell it in the house. Mike opened all the windows, just to satisfy me. He swore that there wasn't even a hint of the odor anywhere. I felt embarrassed for overreacting.

Within the next few days, I began to feel close to human again. While I usually enjoy cooking, I couldn't seem to entertain the thought without a trip to the bathroom. Baking, on the other hand, did appeal to me. I decided to give it a shot. I needed some yeast, so I threw on my coat and ran to the supermarket. As I was leaving the car, I felt a subtle draft on my head. I looked into my rear-view mirror and realized I'd forgotten my scarf. I never wore one at home and was so excited about doing something creative that I forgot to be self-conscious. OK, so here was the test. Would I go in without a scarf, or go home and get it, a total coward. Screw it, I'll go in and give the town something to talk about for the next week.

I walked in and was immediately ridiculed by two useless teenagers who worked there. I just smiled at them, thinking how much money they would save on hair spray if they were bald. It must take an endless supply of spray to get their six inch bangs to stand on end. Who knows how much of the ozone layer has been eliminated for those bangs?

I charged into the milk department where I had difficulty holding back the laughter when the stock boy's doubletake cost him a dozen eggs! I felt like even the frozen peas were staring. I waited in line behind two old women who apparently never graduated from 'Madame Fifi's School of Social Graces.' They were so blatantly obnoxious that I had to quickly think of a way to retaliate.

The first woman struggled to take her change out while her eyes were fixed on me. I finally looked them right in the eyes and said, "Can you believe it, what a bad perm can leave you with, or rather—leave you without?" They were aghast! I left, sure that those two woman would be setting their hair every night for the rest of their lives, rather than risking getting a perm. The good news was I saved them a lot of money. The bread turned out to be worth every minute spent in the market.

"Timidity is a form of vanity. When you are timid, it means that
you attach much more importance to the opinions others have of you
than to the sincerity of your action."

—The Mother
Pondicherry, India

I had to call Donna and tell her about the experience. We both cracked up. It wasn't nearly as funny when it happened as it was when sharing it with other people. Once the laughter died, she said, "Linda, I think I'm going to quit the chemo."

"What? That's ridiculous, Donna. If you quit, who will I have to celebrate with every year in May? Besides, just like me, you made the conscious decision to do this for your life and, damn it, you're gonna do it. There is absolutely no backing down, then wishing you hadn't ten years from now."

"Thanks Linda," she said. "I really needed someone to chew my ass like that!" What I didn't tell her was that I was using the script from the pep talk I had received from Karen just 24 hours earlier.

I had arrived at a crossroads in my decision making. I truly couldn't decide whether or not to have the radiation. I knew Mike wanted me to, but I certainly wouldn't base my decision on his desires. I prayed hard for guidance. My star was nowhere to be seen, so I took it as a sign that I needed to make my pleas known to the Headmaster himself. I asked Cara to pray about it, too.

I awoke to the warm sun shining down through my window, filling my body with new life. I'd nearly forgotten that today was the small treatment day. I got dressed and somberly looked at Mike, "Well I'm going to go through with the radiation for all the right reasons." It puzzled him that I could go to bed with no clue and wake-up totally convinced and at peace with my decision. I'd done the same with the chemotherapy decision. I even told Kai about it, assuring him that he shouldn't experience any side-effects from the radiation. He'd already acquired two small (about the size of a half-dollar) bald patches on his hips. It was almost too much to believe. He hadn't lost any weight and overall, his health seemed to be fine.

I told Diane that I had been experiencing some nasty leg cramps, but nothing intolerable. She said that if it began to interfere with my sleep, she would have a sleeping drug prescribed. I thought, another drug? I didn't think that my body would be able to respond to a mild sleeping pill after all these harsh chemicals but I decided it might be worth a try. I knew sleep was a very important factor in my healing process, so the benefits of taking the medication outweighed my concern about drugs.

I joked around a bit and told her that I thought all my hair was beginning to grow back. Up until now, I had been shaving two small sections on the sides. I thought I would stop after treatment number-five and watch it all grow in! Diane thought it was a great idea and said many woman experienced hair growth before the completion of treatment. I told her that I had access to all the energy in the universe, so it would grow like weeds.

The waiting room was nearly filled today. Everybody appeared to be depressed. For a brief moment, I closed my eyes and pictured myself standing up in front of all these people, shouting, "Today is the first day of eternity! You have been given a chance for spiritual enhancement and advancement. Take this opportunity, utilize it and, I promise, it will bring you to higher places and endless joy!" I must be crazy, I thought. This Kool-Aid was turning me into a *schizo* philosopher. But, I was really enjoying it!

I lay in the bubble-bath and began to think about this disease—or transition process, as I think of it. It was like attending classes at a university, on a pass-fail system. If you pass, you go to a higher plane into what I am certain will be bliss. If you fail, you repeat the class, either in this lifetime or another one. The lesson you missed may be presented to you in an even more difficult manner. I believe that we choose the lessons we'll encounter in our life, like signing up for a curriculum. So you can't see things that happen to you as just bad luck, especially when you have the resources you need to pass. Maybe this is how cancer works. But, how can you be sure that you have graduated in the end? I suppose there really is no definite sign, other than the inner peace we will have finally found.

Everybody is searching for their inner peace, but too many in our society seek it through intellect. Intellect often gets tied up with the ego and interferes with the attainment of peace through ongoing worry and mental competition. You don't have to be smart to attain peace. You need only possess a heart, since that's where the peace is found. I am not saying that I am stupid. But, I accepted God and my spiritual beliefs at such an early age that my intelligence was not a barrier.

During my meditation this morning, I saw my beautiful garden. It grew with incredible speed, with beams of life and beauty. I could smell the aromatic garden and see the wolf watching carefully, so that nothing could threaten it. Again, I began to ponder the ultimate question—what is the proper way to heal the body? This question brought me to an answer that I give my patients. There are many paths to take and a good, better or best system exists for each of us. What might be best for one, will only be good for another.

If we keep open that pure spot in our heart where understanding and truth can be found, the best answer will come to us. Like attracts like, so when you put forth your heart energy, other good energies will begin to gravitate toward you, not through luck, but through natural channels. This is the way nature works, in healing and in all our concerns. Once we understand what our own individual purpose really is on earth, we can draw this to us through the vision in our heart.

Cara had shown no interest in attending any of the chemotherapy sessions. I was hoping, in a strange way, that Cara would decide to come with me for this less hostile treatment. I really wanted, or maybe needed, to share this experience with her. I thought that it would be healthy for her to see me in this environment, surrounded by people who care about me. She'd be able to see that the actual treatment was not so intimidating. To my delight, at the last minute, she decided to go with me. I never pushed the issue of coming with me to a treatment, but I was grateful to be able to share this with her. Mike waited outside through most of it, to allow us some privacy. I decided to invite Meghan to the next appointment.

Today, someone asked me why bad things happen to good people? Since I have never read the book by the same title, I thought for a moment and answered as honestly as I could. First, this doesn't seem to be a very healthy way of looking at such situations. Its not a question of being punished for wrongdoing. When I see a person experiencing trials and tribulations of any kind, I think of it as an opportunity for transition in their life. If we pull our head out of the sand of denial long enough to recognize our mission, we have the potential for gaining great rewards. This brings me back again to why I feel that circumstances are ultimately each person's choice.

A person may turn their entire life around by surviving a minor car accident if they look at the accident as bringing them a message. The message may be, for example, that they are working too many hours, which is why they fell asleep at the wheel. Convalescing at home can show them the love they are missing by being away from their family. These messages may prompt them to change careers or work habits, bringing more love into their life and the lives of their family. On the other hand, they can choose to see it as just a meaningless accident and miss the good it could have done their life.

The message may start with an accident, then a disease, and something after that. Hopefully, you will only get so many taps on the shoulders before you open your eyes wide and say "Oh, I got ya now! The message is loud and clear." Some of us don't receive the message until we are lying on our death bed. I feel this is acceptable too. As long as we get it and come to a full understanding of it so that we may progress upwards.

So, really there is no good or bad, just the message and whether we get it or not. Usually, the difficult part is figuring out what our particular message is and what we need to do about it.

Lately, I have been intrigued by Jeff's transition. He's done so well with this latest breast cancer experience. I felt certain that he'd put his repressed feelings about my mother into a new and healthier perspective. Even his own personal life seems to have gained through this tragedy. With all of the good that has been happening, how could I possibly choose to dwell upon the bad.

I sat down one evening and made a list of the 'good' things and the 'bad' things that had come to light during this period in my life. Some of the bad included catching a draft on my head, vomiting, building up an intolerance to fishes, hand washing my scarves (I despise hand washing!), watching my dog suffer, my veins getting perturbed, and not being able to run. The bad things were obviously inconveniences that would soon pass.

I was amazed at the many meaningful good things! The benefits to Jeff were just the tip of the iceberg. Some others on the list were: the incredible strength I found in my relationship with Mike, seeing more of my friends and family, writing, setting more meaningful life goals, living out my fantasies about being bald, being able to reach out meaningfully and give strength to others during a difficult time, respecting nature in a more profound way, and having the time to knit—something that gives me great pleasure. I spent many loving hours knitting an Icelandic sweater for my chiropractor, Steve, and it felt wonderful to give it to him.

Most of the good things were a result of my mental and spiritual growth and will remain with me forever. This growth showed me that I had been living my life for other people—my clients, my husband and especially my children. I had been trying to be superwoman and make up for all the holes left by my mother's early death. The problem was, those holes were in me, not my daughters. I couldn't fill in *my* holes by over-mothering my daughters and by being the perfect worker. I had to give myself permission to do the things that meant something to me. Filling in the needs left by my mother and rebalancing my relationships allowed me to be a better mother than I could have been before breast cancer. This growth was necessary for me to reach my next step in life.

I know it's been difficult for people who loved and cared for me to watch me through this, but I also know that if they possessed any spiritual depth and they were at all in touch with me, they would realize that I'd be all right. I often wondered where my mother was spiritually before she passed on. The more I learned about her, the more I believed she was, indeed, very spiritual, but maybe lost sight of her intuitions somewhere along the line. I was certain that she came back to them at the end of her life here.

Rummaging through old photographs at least once a year, I always found something new pertaining to Mother's life. My discovery this year was very special. Probably because it answered some of my questions about her spirituality. I found an old piece of index card, with a beautiful, but, somehow, painful message typed on it. I couldn't know for certain whether it was original or not, but I tended to think it was due to the misspelling of words, along with changes made. It read:

> *"It is really something peculiar about the deep in the heart planted homesickness, and also for the longing of distant places. It is no secret, while still at home, we feel more or less the longing for the other place. The yen for "far away" comes alive in us and once far away from home— we feel homesick. We feel not well at all in the country of our choice. We have adjusted ourselves very well, we love our country. And yet, home sickness never leaves us completely, never are we completely*

native. That is the big tragedy in the life of the immigrant. Across in the old home, he is not at home anymore, and here in the country of his choice, deep down in his heart, he is never completely at home. Maybe one should add, where there are children present, whose homeland by nature is here, the so-called tragedy will not be felt quite as strongly. However, it is never absent. We are, at the same time, wanderers, not only between two worlds, but between three worlds, the third being up above, toward which we all strive together."

—Irma Maria Haesicke Phelan

These words made me cry all ten times I read them. I shared it with Jeff. He, too, was deeply touched. I could see she had many repressed feelings about her homeland. I thought she felt she truly belonged there. She always seemed happier there whenever we visited. Reading this brought me close to the pain in her heart. Although she had many friends here, especially ones who shared her love of flying, none were as intimate as her German friends.

Once, I overheard Mother comforting one of her flying students. I don't remember what was bothering her, but I distinctly remembered my mother repeating an old German proverb. Mother told her, "Instead of complaining that the rosebush is full of thorns, be happy that the thorn bush is full of roses." The thought of my Mother possibly being that twinkling star in my window had occurred to me more than once.

My hands were beginning to turn orange from the carrot juice. It was beginning to tweak everyone's curiosity. Aside from being easily fatigued, I was feeling well. I was sure the fatigue was due to the cumulative effect the chemicals were having on my body.

My Sunday for washing out the good old colon was here. The thought of this seemed to give my family an appetite. They all went out for ice cream and had the nerve to brag about it, knowing that I couldn't have any! I began to prepare my insides for the second to the final treatment. It growled for joy.

My counts were fine once again. I had been waiting for someone to ask if there was anything out of the ordinary that I was doing to stay in such good internal health. Today was the day that Dr. Strair asked this question. All along I had been anxious for her to comment on how well I was doing through this so that I could discuss the importance of holistic approaches. Now, for some reason, I would rather wait until my treatments were finished.

We made our way down to the treatment room and I passed the nurse who had guaranteed me that at least one of my treatments would be delayed due to low blood counts. Like a proud punk kid I looked at her and smiled, "Hey, number-five today—and no signs of any delay, hah!" I didn't mean to be arrogant. But, I did want her to realize that not everybody was going to fit into her little "statistical" chart. Some of us would soar above it. After all, there were those of us who were meant to soar and would be damned if we were ever caught doing anything else.

Diane was her usual happy self and the treatment went well. She asked a few times about the girls, so I told her that they would be with me for next week's treatment, that was, if they wanted to. I remember going to one of my mother's treatments. It had been cold and very impersonal. There was absolutely no comparison to the way it was approached these days. We made it down the stairs—and, I had to admit, I was looking forward to walking down them for the very last time.

Mike tucked me into bed as usual. To my wonderful surprise, Beth was there! I managed to give her a hug and talked for all of ten minutes before I knew I had to get to bed and try to fall asleep. It didn't matter. It was just a matter of time before the vomiting began, anyway. This time, I never left the bed. I just kept filling up the bowl for Mike to empty. It was an all-night and all-morning show. I couldn't bring myself to smoke anymore of the 'wonder weed.' I knew the vomiting would pass, and it did. Not as quickly as I would have liked, but it certainly helped knowing that I had only one more treatment to go. I wasn't ready to quit yet. That day, I wrote in my journal, "Higher, always higher! Let us never be still nor satisfied with what we have accomplished."

We had planned a day to visit Kevin and Mary as soon as the weather turned warm. The weather was beginning to break. I could feel spring right around the corner. It made me think of all of the wondrous things that would be happening...all the new life being born, the singing of birds, the overwhelming fragrance of hyacinths and lilacs, and the bright green leaves returning on tall, graceful trees.

Our earth and the animals on it are such a precious resource to me. Nature represents everything beautiful and valuable about being alive. I honestly believe that if we hadn't been born with such powerful minds, we humans would remain directed by nature. Humans have created such havoc in our world's environment. Its not really a question of intelligence as much as ego. Many animals like the dolphin have been proven to have a great deal of intelligence. The dolphin goes to the rescue of its young when they are caught up in fishing nets. There they will stay, comforting their babies until death. Humans are the only creatures on earth who kill and waste animals, like dolphins, that are not food targets.

There was so much to be learned from the Indians if we had just listened instead of killed. They had such a respect for their surroundings and food. They prayed over their kill, thanked the victim for it's nourishment and praised it for it's beauty. They started the day by saying, "Thank you for this beautiful day (regardless of whether it was good or bad), thank you for this life (no matter what kind of life it was), and thank you for the water without which life would be impossible."

The warm day has finally come. As promised, Mary brought out her pottery wheel that I've been eager to play with. Mike and Meg went up to the pond to play with the tadpoles and frogs. Cara hung out with Mary and Maura (their daughter Cara's age) and me. She gave me a crash course in using the wheel, the clay and some of the tools. I was gloriously spinning away.

Obviously—based on the kind of work I do—I love using my hands. To mold something out of earth is something to marvel at. The work made me appreciate the craftsman. Now, when I go to the store and pick up a beautifully crafted bowl, I wonder about the hands that brought the bowl to life, or who put the little dip in the handle. Everything tells a story.

As I watched the clay mold with every command from my hands, I thought just how similar the clay and my body were. They both responded to me. The outcome was a reflection of my thoughts, moods, feelings and emotions. One wrong move and the clay would fall, becoming deformed and out of alignment. If this happens, we must take even more care in bringing it back to center. If it is not precisely on center, the work will be imbalanced. How involved I became with this piece of clay.

Trust was necessary to create a well-centered piece of work...trust in the clay, trust in the wheel and trust within myself. It was not about what I had learned in school or what I would learn in the future, but what I learned from within. The balance I needed was within myself.

This has awakened me to a new analogy of disease. Disease in your body is like what happens to clay when it comes off-center. To become a magnificent work of art, we must find our center. We can, learning from our past errors, forgive ourself for making them and open ourselves to new ideas. Our new balance will provide the kind of environment where disease cannot live.

The stress created by the disease experience is our "firing." Some of us will explode in the kiln and some will develop cracks that refuse to heal. The saddest part is that some of us will survive the firing and refuse to become beautiful porcelain through our own resistance and ignorance. Dealing with this stress can be a truly enlightening experience, just as molding the clay has been. We can smile and even laugh along the way, letting our faith shine through, as well as an occasional tear. And somewhere along the way, pass the hope on to the next person.

It's understandable that disease has gained a bad rap in our society. But, if we could be taught to use disease as a working tool, it has as much potential to create a new life as it does to destroy an old one. And it doesn't stop there...not only does it affect us, but everybody we touch. I pray that I have brought my daughters to a new understanding of the word *cancer*. Even more importantly, I pray they may share the same faith in their lives and forever be aware of staying on a consciously chosen path, careful not to fall astray in unawareness and denial.

Meg graciously accepted my invitation to accompany me to my next treatment. I introduced her to Dr. Strair and Diane. She was a big hit. Dr. Strair gave her a little stuffed dog who was also in for a treatment. She had a little plastic needle and could reenact the entire procedure with her dog. She was very content with this, and I was sure that she could have cared less about watching me. But, when I looked up at her, I noticed she was slyly watching every move Diane made out of the corner of her eye.

When she was satisfied with the evidence that they were not going to hurt me, she decided to walk around the room and introduce herself. There were four elderly people in there at the same time. She went over to every one of them and said, "Hello, my name is Meghan Beth McCoy. I just want you to know that everything is going to be all right. You will be just fine." All the while, she would be stroking their leg while she was talking. Needless to say, they all loved her and were sorry to see her go!

Spring is upon us. The little groundhog should be sticking his head out someday soon. This is fascinating. This little creature of nature knows precisely when to stick his head out to see if it is safe for him to exist outside of his den. Nobody knocks on his door or anything! Thinking about nature and its wondrous activities, I realized that my final chemotherapy treatment is approaching quickly. For some strange reason, I am terrified. I look in the mirror and see a stubbly-headed, freckled-faced little girl. This is the date that I have implanted in my brain, the grand finale. Inside, its similar to the feeling I experienced on my wedding day. I wasn't apprehensive, or sad—but definitely scared shitless. Very much like now, only a week before my treatment.

Being in the office keeps my mind free from the debilitating fear. Watching my stubble grow to a point where it isn't considered stubble anymore is exciting. Its wonderfully freeing not to wear a scarf anymore. I sit and realize just how traumatized my body must be from all the toxins. In another way, I feel taken over by this abundant life force, filled with balanced health and energy. Strange that this could be true. I am very enthusiastic.

> *Happiness isn't really illusive, it's just that we are moving so fast that it has trouble catching up with us!*
>
> —Rosemary

> *There was a time when meadow, grove and stream, The earth and every common sight, to one did seem Apparelled in celestial light, The glory and the freshness of a dream. . . . Our birth is but a sleep and a forgetting: The soul that rises with us, our lifes star, Hath had elsewhere its setting, And cometh from afar: Not in entire forgetfulness, And not in utter nakedness, But, trailing clouds of glory do we come From God, who is our home.*
>
> —William Wordsworth
> "Intimations of Immortality"

The cold bathroom floor grew to be a close friend in the last few weeks. The leg cramping had become almost unbearable at times. I lay on the bathroom floor, hoping the coldness would alleviate it. Once that floor was warm, I went on to the kitchen floor. I gave in and used a few of the sleeping pills, but only in acts of sleep desperation.

I never dreamed that lying there on the floor would feel like an old habit to me, with a plastic tube stuffed up my bum, adjusting the little plastic lever just right, so that the water wouldn't run too fast into me. The entire time, breathing rhythmically to the sounds of the Indian flute music, or following Shakti Gawain's words on visualization.

It seemed almost comical. I remembered Gilda Radner doing skits about having breast cancer. She was hysterically funny. I didn't realize that it was her own way of dealing with her fear of cancer. She was a great person and, I'm sure, continues to be a great spirit, amusing all those other angels and stars up there in the heavens. That's probably why we see the stars twinkle the way they do. They are laughing at one of Gilda's performances.

My body shook the entire way to Providence. I asked Mike to stop so that I could buy some flowers for Diane and Dr. Strair. I knew that I wasn't the most delightful patient all the time, yet they always tolerated me quite well. Now, that deserved an award. I truly appreciated their care. Mike reminded me that I would be coming here regularly for follow-up visits. I resented being reminded of that. He must have seen that by the hairy eyeball I threw him.

The smell of the area nauseated me almost instantly. I couldn't tell if I was overreacting or if I had really debilitated. I was trying hard not to worry about the side-effects since my worrying tended to make things worse. I just had to allow what was going to happen.

Some people tend to be more kinesthetic, relying more on touch, while some are very auditory, relying more on hearing. I am definitely oriented toward the olfactory. My nose knows it all. I smell all my food at restaurants just to make sure it smells right, even at the expense of embarrassing my family. I can remember quite vividly, the smell of the air when we stepped off the plane in Germany. It was one of my favorite smells, because I knew, next, I would be smelling my Oma and her house. I was just a very nosy person!

I met with Dr. Strair and gave her the flowers I had picked out for her. She was moved—but not in the way I was moved every Sunday in my bathroom (...a little sick humor thrown in here). I said, "As long as we were going to be married to each other for the next seventy years, I might as well bring you flowers, like any thoughtful spouse would do!"

She laughed, "Thank you. I apologize for the way you have been feeling all through this awful ordeal, but you are finally there. Your counts have been terrific. So have you. Now, I would like to hear about your secrets for living through this with such ease, compared to other patients."

Dr. Strair continued, "Now I do hope you give yourself a few months before doing any strenuous activity." Yeah, right, I thought silently! It was now my turn to talk. I began with the vitamins. She gave me that familiar look that you get when you try to tell a western-trained physician about holistic medicine—utter skepticism. She was concerned that I had been taking very high doses of the vitamins. I said, absolutely not. I was taking a sufficient amount to help my body repair.

Then, I told her about the enzymes. She, at least, seemed interested in those. I told her about the carrot juice. She was in favor of that. I explained my meditation and visualization. She accepted the idea as most physicians accept it these days. No one was sure why, but too many cases had proven the body-mind connection was important. There were too many good results to just be shunned off as coincidental.

I saved the best for last and explained the colonics. She never blinked an eye. Either she was in total disbelief that she had been treating a woman who made a weekly ritual of sticking a tube up her butt, or because she was actually interested in what I was saying. The latter, I found hard to believe since even Dr. Herman was surprised about this one. He had even made a few cute cracks about it, no pun intended. Great sense of humor, that Dr. Herman has. That's why I love him.

So, I finished my story. She looked at me with sincerity and said, "Hey, it worked for you and that's all I care about." I knew she was not going to run out the door and get her next degree in naturopathic medicine, but, at least, she was open to it and understood that it did indeed make a difference.

Diane almost cried when I gave her the flowers. "I'm so grateful that I got to know you, Linda."

"Not half as grateful as I am for you being here, Diane," I replied. I was sweating before I even hit the chair. "I'm afraid I'm beyond my visualization and breathing techniques. I just feel like swearing right through this one," I said to Mike. He just sat down and squeezed my hand while Diane inserted that awful damn needle for the *last* time. The nausea seemed to take over my entire body. I didn't think I would make it out of there without puking all over the floor. I closed my eyes through the entire treatment. Finally, when it was over, we made it down those despised stairs. *Good riddance*, you ugly gray stairs!

Mike lay me down in the back seat so that I wouldn't lose it in the car. I kept smothering my face in a towel to stop the urge to vomit. At home, I ran through the door and flung open the toilet. I thought it was never going to end. My head felt as though it was being split open from ten different angles. My face was beet red. I honestly thought I was going to die that night.

The violence I experienced could never be put into words. The pain made me feel like slamming my head against a wall. I was up all night and, at one point, I looked in my doorway and saw a figure standing there. I thought it was my guardian angel. "Can I do *anything* to help?" It was Beth. "I can't sleep, I seem to be feeling her headache and nausea," she said to Mike.

"Thanks, Beth," Mike said, "but there really isn't anything to help her right now. I'll call on you if I need a break." By morning, I was still every bit as nauseous. Mike was running all over the place for me. Beth came in and looked at me, helplessly. She so wanted to ease the pain and help in some way.

"Could you please massage my head and neck, Beth?" She smiled and took a gentle hold of my head and just held it for a while. She began wiping my face, neck and chest with a cold wash cloth. I was really burning up. I knew that if this hadn't been the last treatment, I would have made it so. I lay in bed, unable to do anything for the entire day, and the next, and the next. It was taking a long time for me to bounce back from this treatment. It was like the fourth of July fireworks finale exploding in my body. By the fifth day, things began to be tolerable. I could stand the lights around me. My face finally returned to its natural color, which by this time was sort of an ash grey. I was grateful that it was over. It was all behind me. My new life was soon to begin.

I woke up in the morning to the birds singing the songs of life outside the window. I sat on the deck, bundled up in a jacket and blanket, with a cup of tea and lots of hope. Nothing seemed the same to me. It was as though everything alive had been magnified in meaning. I had seen everything here before, yet I was seeing for the first time just how joyous and beautiful life was. I was being intoxicated by the beauty and wildness of every robin and every tree branch. I was sitting in a whirlwind of ecstasy and loveliness of life. We all experienced those magical moments at some point in our life when we were fully aware of the oneness of all things. We could see and understand the processes that were not apparent to us before. This was one of those times for me.

"Peace in the storm, calm in the effort, joy in the surrender, a luminous Faith, and you will become aware of God's constant presence."

— Anonymous

The day for my evaluation at the Auryevedic Health Center in Lancaster, Massachusetts had arrived. I was looking forward to the two-hour drive up there. The weather and the scenery were beautiful on the drive. I never realized how rural this part of New England was. The homes were old and lovely, like something out of a novel. The estate was more elaborate than I had expected. There were a hundred acres of beautiful grounds around the house. It looked like the perfect vacation spot.

I was greeted by a nurse who handed me a health history form to fill out. She mentioned the doctor's name who would be evaluating me, but I had difficulty pronouncing it myself. She was Indian. It took about a half an hour to complete the lengthy form. Then, the doctor presented herself. She was fairly young, about thirty or so, and very beautiful. Her accent was distinct but I had no difficulty understanding her.

We reviewed the health history form and she clarified the areas that seemed vague. The doctor took my pulse, "...very Pitta." I had always known that it was my dominating type. She undressed me and examined my scar and abdomen, along with my eyes, tongue, skin and body. She seemed pleased with what she was seeing, which pleased me. We discussed my past and present diet and she made any necessary additions and eliminations she felt were pertinent. So, the final moment had come.

The doctor said, " You are a healthy young woman and you should expect to live a long and fulfilling life. You have treated the cancer, now accept it as being gone." There were very few changes to make in my diet. She felt I was very much on-track and the important task would be to stay focused. She explained that I should be aware of the subtle symptoms the body and mind may display when it began to fall off-track, and how to bring it back into harmony. Overall, it was very satisfying experience. I was happy I decided to go. I ordered the herbs and some of the seasonings which I find extremely palatable and fun to cook with.

I agreed to return in the future for a simple follow-up appointment. She supported having the radiation therapy. I knew she herself was a radiologist and asked if this was why she agreed. She replied, no. She sincerely felt that I should not stop halfway. "You should see the treatments through," she said. I could do that, I thought to myself.

CHAPTER 11

THE ELECTRIC BEACH

I arrived at Dr. Masko's office early to discuss the radiation treatment. She explained that the silicone implants posed no threat to either me or to the treatments. I would be seen daily, five times a week, for six weeks. The sixth week, I would be sent to Rhode Island Hospital where they had a specific type of machine to give me a boost in selected areas...the armpit and the large tumor site. I was not to use any lotions, powders, or deodorant during those six weeks because of the radiation. The skin would become irritated and itchy. A big emphasis was put on not scratching any itching places.

My blood work would be done weekly to watch my white cell count. It would not alter them to the degree of chemotherapy but it would make them drop some. There would be one long appointment in the beginning called the assimilation, or 'marking' appointment. That was when all the measurements would be done and I would be marked with tiny little tattoos, enabling the technician to precisely set the machine. I agreed to it all and made the assimilation appointment for two days later.

For the next two days, I made all the necessary adjustments in my schedule to accommodate going for radiation every morning at eight-thirty. I estimated when the treatments would be ending. It should be the first week of July.

The assimilation appointment turned out to be a real test of patience. I lay on a large table with my right arm up over my head, grasping a handle. This was a difficult position for anyone after having a mastectomy. After about five minutes of this position, my arm began to fall asleep, the most irritating sensation. Of course, it was extremely important that I did not move during this procedure, or it would have to be repeated from the beginning. I asked, "What do they do with little old ladies having to lay in this position for over an hour?"

"We do all we can—and that is to wipe their tears." How dreadful I thought. I tried to figure out another way they could measure accurately without as much discomfort and without risking the end result. The only thing I could come up with was to extend the arm back as far as it would go and then at least rest a pillow under it for some support.

The radiation treatments began on a Monday. My blood counts were beginning to come back up, but they told me my blood wouldn't really recover until the radiation was over. My technician, Patty, was a sweetie. I took an immediate liking to her. I enjoyed talking to her even though our conversations were brief—because the actual treatments took all of ten minutes.

The traffic was so unpredictable that, many times, I arrived fifteen minutes early. The table was as large as the table where I was measured. They strapped me onto it and again I had to hold my arm over my head and turn my face to the left. The noise from the machine was loud and obnoxious. It was difficult to relax during the procedure because of this.

I would close my eyes and go into a meditative, restful and alert state. I repeated, again and again, "The healing light is surrounding my body." I was amazed at how relaxed I was when it was time for me to get off the table. I felt as though I had meditated for twenty minutes. The feeling was profound.

Everyday, Patty asked, "How is your progress rebounding from bodily chemical warfare?"

"Always getting better," I'd say, and then we'd laugh. Mike never came to any of these treatments. I think he was doing his own rebounding and regrouping. Beth came out for a visit and was allowed to come into the room with Patty and me.

When I got off the table, I looked at her, and she at me and we both cried. I realized we'd never cried together, though she'd spent a lot of time around me at my worst. It was nice to go for coffee and just talk with her. It was very difficult for her to see me in such a vulnerable position, but she was grateful for the experience and for me allowing her to share it. I was sure she'd never know just how much she gave to me in those times. I felt the same about the many other friends and family members who stood by me in those tough times. I was a very lucky person to be woven into a web of such beautiful beings.

I met Dr. Masko in the hospital for the new measurements and to be introduced. The itching and burning had been minimal. The technicians insisted on marking me with new tattoos even though they had already colored me in, like a coloring book, with a magic marker. I refused the tattoos and promised I wouldn't wash off the marker.

This wasn't like being with Patty. My new technician was abrasive and extremely unprofessional. She was smacking her gum all the while she was leaning over my face measuring. I thought I would scream when I felt the spit coming out of her mouth. She was using a metal ruler to take the measurements which was not a smart thing to do. She turned around abruptly and nearly took my silicone out with no anesthesia! I was not a happy camper. I left in total disgust, but decided that I would give it another chance.

The second treatment turned out to be as unbelievable as the first. I lay on the table feeling desperate and destitute. No more, I thought to myself. This was the completion of my treatment. I went home and very calmly phoned Dr. Masko and said, "Look, I have really given this a shot and can't go back there again. They're the most unprofessional, inconsiderate people I have ever been in the company of." She said, "OK, I understand. You are not the first person to make that complaint, but I'm satisfied with the amount of radiation you have received. Would you mind terribly sending the administrator of the hospital a letter explaining your experience?"

"Absolutely not," I said. "I have every intention of making myself heard." I hung up the phone and it hit me. It was over! Really over! I phoned Mike and we agreed to celebrate with a Tito Burrito. I ran my fingers through my one and a half inch hair and fell back onto the bed with a sigh of accomplishment!

CHAPTER 12

THE JOURNEY COMPLETE:
CELEBRATION OF LIFE IN THE HIGHER PLACES

The radiation ended on a Friday, so we declared Monday a day of celebration. The Steve Winwood concert I had so long anticipated was here in time to celebrate! Since Mike was not a *true* Winwood fan, he insisted I invite a friend who I knew enjoyed the performer. I invited Carolyn, the only person I knew who could still live life at one-hundred miles per hour and still raise two children. Her energy made her great fun to be around.

My brother, Jeff, bought us a limousine ride to mark this very special time in my life. We stood up out of the moon roof while going over the Mount Hope bridge and popped the champagne cork! The concert was fabulous. We had reach-out-and-touch-him seats, and it was all I could do to contain myself from doing just that. We danced until we couldn't dance any longer. It was a wonderful celebration!

I had been looking forward to Rosemary's visit, hoping that all the stubble would be covering my head and it did. It added to the reward of the visit. In great anticipation, we'd made several plans for celebrating life together. The most special one was a trip on a whale-watch boat. We almost missed it by getting lost on the way out there, but as it turned out we could get on the next boat. We sucked in our breath at the first spotting of a whale. And then, there was another and another. It was endless! We were all speechless, witnessing the splendor of those beautiful creatures. They were so large yet so graceful.

Meghan stuck to her Auntie like glue and I could see she was well accepted. Rosemary and I had nights to chat and spent some time together which was always a great pleasure. It was wonderful for Cara. She seemed to really enjoy having her Aunt around for girl-chat. It was very interesting to listen to Rosemary talk about the girls. She only saw them periodically, so their growth and maturity were more evident to her. She saw each stage from a different perspective than I, their mother.

Convinced that Dr. Barrall likes to gloat over his beautiful handiwork, I faithfully attended my next appointment. We sat down and he said, "Well, now that the radiation is completed, we can go ahead and do it."

"I beg your pardon?"

"Well haven't we discussed nipples?"

"Not in this life." So he described the nipple procedure. I was the perfect little considerate patient, allowing him to finish all he had to say. I had come to the conclusion that plastic surgeons were like artists. They were not only perfectionists, but they had to get their signature on every piece of work. This was what the nipples were to Dr. Barrall.

So now it was my turn and I think he was surprised by what I had to say. "Dr. Barrall, why would I want to put myself through another surgery at this time? First of all, I have no need for nipples. I am not a stripper. Secondly, do you know what fun it can be going to the market these days? Every time I have to hang over the frozen food section, I look up to see some poor baffled, pathetic man wondering what the heck is wrong with me! The smooth look is in!"

Obviously, Dr. Barrall had never been told "no" on nipples with this sort of an explanation. Finally, he snapped to look at me and said, "That's one way of putting it!" I promised he would be the first to know if I ever changed my mind.

I thanked him from the bottom of my heart and gave him a beautiful flowering cactus. He was so appreciative. I said, "I'll give you a few more years in private practice. You'll not only be a great patient hugger, but you'll also have a greenhouse full of plants." I drove home with a smile on my face, smiling at everyone who passed me. The day was filled with splendor and was topped off by a telephone call from Debbie sharing her joyful news that she was pregnant!

The week was full of publicity. I found myself picking up the newspaper and reading the continuing saga of silicone implants. I suppose women are justified in directing their anger toward the company. But, I also think these women should take some responsibility for what they choose to have put into their bodies. Especially women who had them implanted for purely aesthetic reasons.

Personally, I chose to have the implants, fully acknowledging the fact that they could pose a problem in the future. And I wouldn't part with them for all the tea in China! I did refuse to have nipples put on, but, as I explained to Dr. Barrall, it left some creativity for me and Mike. At Christmas time, we can color in little Santas and on Valentine's Day, little hearts. How clever!

I suppose the bottom line to all of the silicone controversy is that the companies will now be forced to provide women with a safer product, with no health risks involved. Of course, this would be great. As the days passed, I realized that I no longer looked at my breasts as being foreign or as not belonging. I could pass myself naked in the mirror and my stare no longer rested on my chest. My breasts were truly a part of me.

Then, I turned the page to read the latest news on Magic Johnson. I'll never forget sitting in front of the television, just a week ago, and hearing CNN release the news that shocked the sports world—Magic has the HIV virus. Many people were diagnosed with this dreaded disease but no one would have predicted Magic to be one of them. My heart went out to him.

I knew Mike was on his way home and I hoped that he wouldn't hear it then. Magic's retirement announcement was due to be televised that evening and I knew that we would be glued to the television watching it. Mike walked in the door with a somber look on his face. I knew he had taken it very hard. We sat in front of the TV together and respectfully listened to Magic's announcement. It reminded me of Nixon's resignation. My parents had sat in front of our television, just as we did, with that same saddened, somber look upon their faces.

Even the girls were silent, out of respect. Although Meg was not aware of the full impact of Magic's illness, she was still sympathetic. She even made him a get well picture and we sent an inspirational card thanking him for the joy and excitement he had given us, especially that day in Boston. It just proved that life was full of uncertainties. But, we must not dwell upon tomorrow, we must live today to its fullest.

"But, let every man prove his own work, and then shall he have rejoicing in himself alone, and not in another"

—Galatians 6:4

We are now the proud and nervous parents of a high school teenager. My goodness, will the house ever be the same? She has chosen public high school, tried out and made the varsity soccer team. We are beaming!

Meg is the proud first-grader. I still cannot believe that an entire year has passed since my diagnosis. So much has happened. So much has changed. I suppose this will always be the case in the house of the McCoy's. I suppose we should always have our faces toward change and behave like the free spirits we truly are. Truly.

I have begun my running schedule. Mike is so concerned that I may drop dead of heart failure that he has decided to take up running with me. I'm certain this won't last. Even though he has the perfect build to run— very streamlined and virtually no hips—he swears he'll never do it. He always watches runners and points out how miserable they look. I guess he has never watched himself play racquetball. Well, I could barely make it to the end of our housing development. The only reason I made it that far was because the girls had just gotten on the bus and it was coming down the street and I was not about to get razzed by Cara for not being able to run a hundred yards. Talk about stubborn pride.

I kept at it at least three times a week and, within three weeks, I could jog the three-mile course without stopping. I was jogging though, not running. It was taking me twelve minutes to do one mile, but hey, I can live with that...for about three more weeks, maybe. I am not looking for running to become a dreary habit for me. I enjoy it too much for that. I don't believe any part of life should be just a habit. It should always be fresh with excitement and marvel, making us eager and satisfied to live in every moment.

November is here and I am shocked to realize it is my one-year anniversary with breast cancer. This brings to the surface some loaded emotions. I say loaded because however you choose to deal with them will decide whether you sink or swim. I have much more respect for life along with a new and intimate sense of mortality. I still spend time with

Donna and we share a lot of feelings with each other. It's nice to have somebody to bounce ideas and complaints off of. I am sure we will be lifelong friends. She is a beautiful person, indeed.

I am working with many ex-cancer patients these days. They tell me that I bring them new hope. My outlook on life and living has a tendency to be catching. They like this. But, they also seem to be interested in what I have to say about death and dying. I have never had a morbid outlook on death. It bewilders me that some people feel this way. I think the people who believe that the only death they will ever experience is a physical death have a much greater acceptance of it.

It is Thanksgiving, once again. The thanks and praise runneth over at our dinner table. Not only for being together and healthy, but for the smaller things, too, like being able to run eight-and a-half-minute miles— finally. Thank you, God!

Today, I am honored with the privilege of being part of a welcoming party. Not just any party. I have been asked to participate in the labor and delivery of Debbie's first child. To witness the splendor of a new life entering into the world gives a feeling that no words can convey. A new, tiny, miraculous life. I look into little Nicholas's face and ask, "Who are you?" It truly is a miracle. Happy birthday, little person! The day gives me an opportunity to remember that life itself is a wondrous gift.

Maybe his spirit was resting up in the heavens, twinkling in someone's window, before it entered into the world! I am sure that I, too, will be called upon someday to twinkle in the night sky in the corner of someone's window to fill them with hope and peace. But, for now, I will continue to be an instrument, chosen by my creator, to play in his band of light.

> *The peace of the running wave to you,*
> *The peace of the flowing air to you,*
> *The peace of the quiet earth to you, and*
> *The peace of the shining stars to you...*
> *And the peace of the son of Peace to you.*

> —a Celtic benediction (anonymous)

AND THERE WILL ALWAYS BE A SEASON FOR ME...

Epilogue

I began my struggle with breast cancer in the Autumn. This was fortunate for me. It meant that the timing of my treatment and recovery would mirror my sense of nature and her timing. Since I was a child, Autumn has been my favorite time of year. Through those years of early childhood and eventually, adolescence and maturity, I began to refer to Autumn as my high-energy time. A time when my life's mishaps and falls have a seemingly effortless ability to come back together to a graceful balance.

As I began the process of healing, I saw myself following the natural transition made by the living world around me. I lost my leaves, became dormant, and awoke to a spring of new life. My exterior coverings changed tremendously while my core stayed the same. Having for so long admired the beauty of this process, I could easily accept my place within it. I believe that this acceptance was my key to recovery.

As beautiful as the New England autumn is, not everyone has the same love for it. Most New Englander's are focused on the unkind winter to follow. Some say it reminds them of death and dying. Most of the people I speak to with cancer seem to regard this disease in the same way, as a dying process. I'd like to help them to see it differently.

What they are failing to see is that cancer, like Autumn, begins the clearing away of the old before the new can blossom. It's a time of transition. And if we were not so far astray from mother nature herself we'd be conscious of this time and use it to accomplish the same thing. Just like the earth, we must become silent and inward to hear and gain the most from the transformation.

I have learned many different lessons from this disease. But, above all, the experience has reinforced my innate belief that as a part of the natural physical world we need to embrace our place in nature. Nature is so beautifully simple. For us to regain our simplicity, we must begin with restoring the nature in us. By this, I mean we must bring our *self* back to our most balanced and uncomplicated form mentally, physically and spiritually.

I believe that there is one unified theory for all creation. We are here for a reason, but in order to stay, we must first make a commitment. We must give as much meaning to our lives as we possibly can. It's here that health can reside.

On the following pages are some of my suggestions I call *Feel Goods*, for helping you to rebalance your inner self while you heal your outer self. I have also included a reading list of the books which have helped me on my path. I send you my love and best wishes for finding the way along your path.

Appendix

FEEL GOODS

- Get up in the morning and give yourself a massage using a light sesame oil and don't leave out any body parts, including your head and face. What a great way to bring love of your *self* into your self, as well as to explore your new body.

- Practice lying in the bathtub (best done while you're alone in the house!) and relaxing your jaw so that it hangs all the way open. Now relax every muscle in your body and take a breath in. On the exhale, let *any* noise come out that wants to. If it sounds musical and pretty, you are not doing this exercise correctly. Let it be honest, no matter how awful it sounds. It may take a while to get used to it, but it will begin to feel like an incredible release!

- Every day, find something of nature. Seek the uniqueness and wonder about it. Example, the miraculous way a flower begins to emerge from a bud, or the intricate pattern of moss growing in the woods.

- Have someone read to you. Even children!

- Collect as many hugs as possible in the course of a day.

- Pose naked in front of a mirror every day and remind yourself just how beautiful you are. If this is too much, try lighting a candle in a dark room with a mirror. It is more subtle.

- Use a self-tanning cream and pretend you've been on vacation. I used one by Origins. It has infusions of sage (great for negative emotion cleansing), winterbloom and other wonderful herbs.

- Get a massage by a licensed therapist once a week, or as often as you can afford it.

- Learn to meditate. A little yoga wouldn't hurt. And no, you don't have to be pencil thin and rubbery to do it. Yoga is more importantly about proper breathing and freeing your mind. Aaaaah...!

- Be outrageous when you want to be. People will get over it. Just don't hurt anyone in the process, including yourself.

- Grow a little herb garden in your kitchen window. You can use them or just enjoy them in the dirt.

- Take pictures of nature to remind yourself that you are a part of the whole scheme of things, and you *do* matter.

- Draw, paint, play with clay, howl at the moon, whatever it takes to let go of the fear.

SUGGESTED READING

Minding the Body, Mending the Mind by Joan Boryensenko, Ph.D.

Quantum Healing by Dr. Deepak Chopra

The Woman's Comfort Book by Jennifer Louden

Dr. Susan Love's Breast Book by Dr. Susan Love

The Magic of Touch by Sherry Suib Cohen

The Breast Cancer Journal by Juliet Wittman

Anatomy of an Illness by Norman Cousins

The Alexander Technique by Judith Leibowitz and Bill Connington

When I am An Old Woman I Shall Wear Purple edited by Sandra Martz

Angel Wisdom by Terry Lynn Taylor and Mary Beth Crain

Breathing Into Life by Bija Bennett

Colon Health by Norman Walker, M.D.

Mediation, The Eight Point Program by Eknath Easwarn Nigri Press